101 AMAZING USES for

HONEY

Published by Familius LLC, www.familius.com

Familius books are available at special discounts for bulk purchases, whether for sales promotions or for family or corporate use. For more information, contact Familius Sales at 559-876-2170 or email orders@familius.com.

Library of Congress Cataloging-in-Publication Data
2018937189

Print ISBN 9781641700443
Ebook ISBN 9781641700955

Printed in the United States of America

Edited by Laurie Duersch
Cover design by David Miles
Book design by Caroline Larsen

10 9 8 7 6 5 4 3 2 1

First Edition

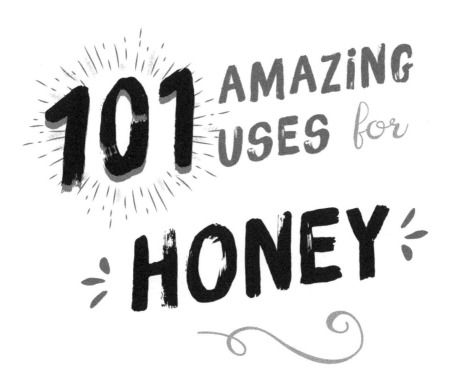

101 AMAZING USES for HONEY

CLEAN SCRAPES & CUTS,
SOFTEN YOUR SKIN,
MAKE A SOOTHING BATH,
AND 98 MORE!

Susan Branson

CONTENTS

CHAPTER 2: SAFEGUARD WELL-BEING I 55

CHAPTER 3: SALVAGE HAIR AND SKIN | 105

CHAPTER 4: INDOORS AND OUTDOORS | 121

NOTES | 139

INTRODUCTION

HONEY AND WHY IT SHOULD BE A STAPLE IN YOUR PANTRY

Honey is a thick, golden liquid that is found in almost any grocery store. Fresh, local honey is often readily available at farmer's markets and roadside stands, or from beekeepers themselves.

There are over three hundred varieties of honey in the United States, each with its own color and flavor profile. These unique properties are derived from the particular sugary liquid (nectar) gathered from each plant. Hardworking honeybees travel from one plant to another and extract the nectar from flowers using their long tongues. They store the liquid in their stomachs, where it mixes with enzymes. They then fly back to their hive, where they regurgitate the nectar into a waiting honeybee's mouth. This bee ingests and regurgitates the nectar many more times until it is ready to be stored in a honeycomb. While here, most of the water is evaporated from the honey. Bees then seal the honey with beeswax to preserve it as a future food source.

Beekeepers, on the other hand, remove the honeycombs with the honey before sealing. The resulting raw product is ready to be consumed. Proper storage in sealed sterile containers can preserve honey indefinitely.

Honey contains sixty-four calories in one tablespoon and is 25 percent sweeter than table sugar. Unlike sugar, raw honey will not cause a spike in blood sugar and a rise in insulin. It is made up mostly of sugars, but it also contains amino acids, vitamins, minerals, enzymes, and a multitude of phytochemicals. The amount of each of these depends on the flower, the season, and the region from which the nectar was sourced. How the honey was harvested, processed, and stored also affects the final composition.

Darker honey can have up to twenty times the antioxidant potential of lighter honeys. Antioxidant activity is just one of the many bioactive roles honey plays. Honey is antimicrobial and anti-inflammatory. It can heal wounds, improve cardiovascular conditions, prevent infection, diminish tumor growth, reduce glucose levels, and even help manage weight. It can be consumed or put on the skin. It can be used for its nutritional value or for its therapeutic benefit.

Honey's importance is ever increasing, and the reputation of honey will continue to rise as more studies emerge to shine light on its expanding and considerable capacity to heal, strengthen, and rejuvenate.

....

HONEY: DISCOVERY AND USES

Bees have been making honey for countless ages, and man likely discovered this sweet liquid and used it in their diet long before historical evidence indicates.

Stone Age paintings show the use of honey over eight thousand years ago, and beeswax in pottery and cooking pots indicates that honey was consumed regularly. Other cultures regarded honey highly in their diet, medical practices, and beauty routines. The Egyptians had beekeepers who used hardened mud pots or hollow logs hung from trees as beehives. They collected the honey and used much of it in their medicines, including a salve for wound healing. The Greeks drank a beverage made from honey and unfermented grape juice for nervous disorders. The famed Greek physician Hippocrates prescribed honey and vinegar for pain and used honey in a variety of other remedies, including those for sore throats, coughs, and eye diseases. Ayurvedic medicine, one of the world's oldest medical systems that originated in India, considered honey a gift to mankind. It promoted honey for those with weak digestion, coughs, insomnia, unhealthy gums and teeth, cardiovascular issues, eye ailments, and skin disorders.

The religious significance of honey is prominent throughout history. Egyptians buried honeycombs in the tombs of pharaohs—it was still edible upon recent discovery—and used honey in embalming their dead. Buddhists in India and Bangladesh give honey to monks during the Honey-Offering Festival. This honors the legend of a monkey's offering of honey to Lord Buddha when he retreated into the wilderness to bring peace to his disciples. The Hindus believe honey is one of five remedies for immortality and pour it over the statues of deities in one of their rituals. Jewish New Year celebrations involve dipping apple slices in honey to symbolize a sweet and fruitful new year.

Today, honey is consumed as a sweetener and is often advocated as a healthier alternative to sugar. More and more people are becoming aware of honey's therapeutic value and are including a little honey a day into their diets for its nutritional components: antioxidants, minerals, amino acids, vitamins, and enzymes.

The constantly emerging scientific studies are validating what centuries of our predecessors have known—honey is a functional food that can be used every day to improve a wide array of medical issues, inside and out. It can improve our mental and physical well-being, all the while masquerading as a key ingredient in sweet confections.

IS HONEY SAFE FOR ME?

The chemical makeup of honey depends on which plants the bees extract their nectar from. Some plants may be contaminated with microorganisms, which would transfer to the honey. Dust and germs can also mix with the honey during the production, processing, and distribution processes. Typically, the antimicrobial activity of the honey prevents the survival of these organisms.

One exception is bacteria that form spores and release a toxin that may cause botulism (a rare but very serious form of food poisoning). This is potentially fatal in babies and young children and is the reason why **raw honey should never be given to infants orally before they reach the age of one**. Single appropriate doses of honey can be safely administered to children older than twelve months. Speak with your doctor before giving raw honey to a young child with immune-deficiency issues.

Oral consumption of honey produced from the rhododendron flower (called "mad honey") should also be avoided by all age groups. This contains grayanotoxin, a compound that may cause poisoning and lead to serious cardiovascular symptoms.

A few things to be aware of is that all types of honey lengthen blood-clotting time and may increase bleeding when used alongside antiplatelet or anticoagulant drugs, supplements, or herbs; this includes aspirin, nonsteroidal anti-inflammatories, warfarin, heparin, garlic, ginger, clove, ginkgo, and others. Sometimes honey can cause allergic reactions, stinging of the nasal passages if used intranasally, or nausea, vomiting, or stomachache. Some children are susceptible to hyperactive behavior, nervousness, or insomnia.

Otherwise, honey is deemed likely safe in children and adults, including pregnant women. This includes both topical application and internal ingestion, when used in appropriate amounts.

HOW MUCH HONEY IS TOO MUCH?

It's difficult to overdo it with honey. For most, the sweet taste and thick texture tend to satisfy cravings rather quickly, making over-indulgence less of a possibility.

Whether administration is oral or topical, the honey used should be raw, unprocessed honey or medical-grade honey to be most effective. The latter has been irradiated with gamma rays to inactivate bacterial spores to prevent the ingestion of toxins that may cause poisoning, like botulism. Medical-grade honey has also been standardized to contain consistent levels of antibacterial potency.

Ayurvedic medicine recommends consuming no more than four to five teaspoons of honey each day. Therapeutic doses tend to be higher and depend on the weight of the individual, as well as the ailment being treated. As a general estimate, between seven and ten teaspoons are generally recommended each day for adults. These should be equally divided throughout the day. Children's doses also vary according to their weight and typically range anywhere from half a teaspoon to several teaspoons a day, depending on the complaint.

Topically, honey can be applied on dressings or directly to wounds for as long as needed. They can be changed twice daily, every other day, or every week.

THE MANY TYPES OF HONEY

There are hundreds and hundreds of different types of honey made by honeybees, each unique in flavor, color, and medicinal qualities. The type of flower that the bees use to collect their nectar dictates these characteristics.

Nectar from buckwheat is dark and full-bodied, high in iron and antioxidants, and bold in taste. At the other end of the spectrum is acacia honey. This is light in color with a very sweet, mild floral flavor. It is high in fructose and low in sucrose (sugar), making it a good choice for diabetics.

Some honeys are made from just one type of flower, called mono-floral honey, while others are made from multiple flowers and are referred to as polyfloral. The amounts and types of vitamins, minerals, and phytochemicals in honey depend on the plants used by the bees. The nectar collected contains all the benefits of the plant. Plants high in antioxidants will have nectar high in antioxidants. Plants that have elevated antibacterial compounds will pass those into the nectar as well.

One type of honey that has become very popular over the past several years is manuka honey. This monofloral honey is only made in New Zealand where bees extract nectar from the manuka bush. Interestingly, this tree is related to the tree from which the potent antibacterial tea tree oil originates. Manuka honey has much higher concentrations of minerals than other types of honey and superior antibacterial levels. In fact, the purity and quality of manuka honey is standardized and reported by a UMF, unique manuka factor. This is essentially a grading system developed by the UMF Honey Association in New Zealand. When buying this honey, choose a manuka honey that has a UMF10+. This means that it is of high quality and has therapeutic levels of antimicrobial compounds. UMF16+ is considered superior quality. Medical-grade, sterilized manuka UMF honey is now approved for use in wound dressings, ointments, and gels in the United States, Canada, Europe, New Zealand, Australia, and Hong Kong. The honey is irradiated to inactivate any bacterial spores but still retains its anti-microbial activity.

Honey can be purchased both in raw and processed forms. Raw honey is crude honey collected from the honeycomb that contains a number of impurities like bees, wings, legs, and beeswax, among other things. The honey is strained to remove these components. The thick, opaque liquid is then bottled.

Processed honey is filtered and pasteurized to destroy micro-organisms with heat and remove them from the honey. Most honey is heated above 145 degrees Fahrenheit (63 degrees Celsius), a temperature that destroys nutrients, antioxidants, and antimicrobial compounds. The resulting honey is golden, clear, and syrup-like. Often, additives are mixed with the honey. Some contain high fructose corn syrup, known to increase the risk of a variety of health problems like diabetes and cardiovascular issues. Processed honey can also be sourced from poorly nourished bees treated with antibiotics or hives made from nonorganic materials that may not be properly sterilized.

CHAPTER 1

SUPPORT HEALTH OVER DISEASE

HEALTH

WELL-BEING

BEAUTY

HOME

1. ASTHMA

Asthma is a chronic condition in which the airways leading to the lungs are inflamed. When exposed to triggers (chemicals or situations that impact the body), the airways swell and produce extra mucus. The passageway for air narrows and breathing becomes more difficult. Symptoms include coughing, shortness of breath, wheezing, and chest pain.

Anyone can develop asthma, although some are genetically predisposed to it. Triggers can be allergens (from the environment or from food) or other substances like smoke, pollution, or changes in the weather. Learning what your specific triggers are goes a long way in asthma management. Doctors often prescribe controller medications like corticosteroids (cortisone-like medications used to provide relief), long-acting beta agonists, and sometimes leukotriene modifiers to help manage the condition. Short-acting beta agonists are prescribed to quickly relieve symptoms by relaxing and opening the airways.

Because of the increasing and alarming rise of asthma in children and adults, it is more important than ever to find ways to manage this condition without the overuse of controller medications. Ayurvedic medicine has a recipe for preventing asthma attacks that includes consuming a mixture of honey, ginger juice, and black pepper powder with a recommended dosage of three times a day.

Parents of asthmatic children in some countries rely heavily on complementary and alternative medicine to help their children cope with this condition. In Istanbul, Turkey, a study found

41.6 percent of patients using alternative therapies chose honey to manage their asthma.[1] They may be on to something. Rabbits with asthma given aerosolized honey had reduced mucus production and fewer inflammatory cells in their lung fluid.[2] These results indicate honey may show promise in the treatment of asthma in humans.

2. BREAST CANCER

Breast cancer starts when cells of the breast begin to grow out of control and form a tumor. Tumors are cancerous if they grow and spread into other areas of the body. The condition is much more common in women, but men can develop breast cancer too. Mammograms can help detect the cancer before symptoms begin. If not detected early, breast cancer can cause bloody discharge from the nipple or changes in the shape or texture of the breast or nipple. It can also be felt as a lump. Treatment may involve radiation, chemotherapy, or surgery.

This is the most common cancer among women, so finding new and effective therapies is critical to help increase survival rates. Tualang honey (wild honey from the rainforests of Malaysia) was found to be cytotoxic to human breast cancer cells. A normal breast cell line tested concurrently was not affected.[3] This honey also promotes the anticancer activity of tamoxifen, a drug used to prevent or treat breast cancer.[4] When taken together, tualang honey has the potential to reduce tamoxifen dosage and its side effects. Results in live rats with induced breast cancer showed that four months of tualang honey treatment reduced the incidence, progression, size, mass, and weight of tumors compared to rats that did not receive any honey.[5]

Manuka honey from New Zealand also boasts anticancer activity. It activates a metabolic cell pathway that leads to DNA fragmentation and cell death of the cancer cells. Manuka honey destroyed breast cancer cells in a time- and dose-dependent manner.[6] This again highlights the use of honey with traditional cancer drugs to reduce drug dosage and lower the risk of side effects.

3. CANDIDIASIS

Candidiasis is a fungal infection caused by the yeast-like *Candida* fungus. There are over twenty species of *Candida* that can infect humans, but *Candida albicans* is the most common.

These yeasts normally live on the skin and mucous membranes in people and are generally harmless. If conditions in the body shift to create an environment favorable to *Candida* overgrowth, infections of the mouth, vagina, urinary tract, skin, or stomach can set in. Most causes of *Candida* overgrowth result from certain drugs, pregnancy, bacterial infections, excess weight, or an overburdened immune system. Vaginal yeast infections, white lesions on the tongue or inner cheek, painful cracks in the skin at the corners of the mouth, or crusted skin rashes around the fingers, toes, and groin are symptoms of candidiasis.

Antifungal drugs are commonly prescribed for up to two weeks. Reducing sugar and yeast products in the diet and taking probiotics are popular complementary approaches to assist in eliminating candidiasis.

Honey is able to inhibit the growth of *Candida*[7] and can be consumed internally, applied topically on the skin, or diluted with warm water and swished around the mouth.

When *Candida* forms biofilms, it can be extremely difficult to treat. This is when the cells become embedded in an extracellular matrix and stick to each other and other surfaces. They are often antibiotic resistant, can evade the body's natural defenses, and frequently lead to chronic infections. Jujube honey can be used in these cases to disrupt the structure of mature biofilms and decrease their thickness. This honey can also be used to inhibit the formation of new biofilms and prevent chronic infections.[8]

4. CATHETER-RELATED INFECTIONS

Catheters are soft tubes made from thin silicone, rubber, vinyl, or plastic that deliver or remove fluids to or from the body.

In people with kidney disease, catheters are one of the ways to access and clean the blood and remove extra fluid from the body; the kidneys are not able to adequately perform these functions on their own. The catheter is placed under the skin of the neck and must be kept clean and dry to prevent infection; however, the surface of the catheter often becomes coated with plasma proteins, which attracts bacteria and fungi from the skin. These can grow at the exit site of the catheter and get into the bloodstream, causing a bloodstream infection. The body's immune response to this infection may lead to septic shock, which could be fatal.

Some of the bacteria that form at the catheter's exit site are antibiotic resistant and hard to control. Antiseptic agents like mupirocin are effective at killing many of these germs, but some continue to thrive. In addition, antibiotic ointments have unpleasant side effects in some people, including diarrhea and stinging at the application site. In a study, Medihoney, a wound dressing made from manuka honey, was applied three times a week in patients receiving hemodialysis by venous catheters. It was found to be as effective as mupirocin in reducing exit-site infections and bloodstream infections. The honey was also more successful fighting against antibiotic-resistant microorganisms than mupirocin.[9] Honey proved to be not only effective but also a safer and cheaper alternative to antibiotic drugs.

5. CERVICAL CANCER

Cells of the cervix may gradually begin to develop precancerous changes. These changes can be detected by a Pap smear and treated so that they do not progress into cancerous cells. While not all precancerous cells develop into cancer if left alone, those that do become cancerous often take a few years to make the actual change to cancer cells.

Cancer cells multiply uncontrollably and do not die as normal, healthy cells do. They form into masses called tumors, which can break off and spread to other areas of the body. One of the causes of cervical cancer is human papillomavirus, or HPV. There are various types of this virus, and it is quite common. It is contracted by having sex with an infected person, even if the carrier shows no signs or symptoms. Most cases of HPV resolve on their own, but some will develop into cervical cancer. Lifestyle factors like smoking may also increase the risk of developing cervical cancer. Treatment depends on how far the cancer has progressed. In the early stages, surgery to remove the cervix and uterus (along with perhaps the lymph nodes and part of the vagina) often removes the cancer. Others opt for radiation and chemotherapy to shrink tumors and kill cancer cells. Those in the later stages of this cancer often combine radiation with chemotherapy.

Tualang honey from the rainforests of Malaysia has been investigated as an anticancer agent in cervical cancer. Cervical cancer cell lines were treated with tualang honey for up to three days, in increasing doses. All the cancerous cells were destroyed. Mitochondrial function, a key indicator of the health of the cell, was reduced and the pathway to destroy the malignant cells was activated. Cellular contents were observed leaking through the cell membrane, resulting in cell death.[10] **Healthy, normal cells were not affected by the honey.** Other honey may have this anticancer potential as well and can be used with doctor-prescribed treatments in the fight against cervical cancer.

6. CHICKEN POX

Chicken pox is a viral infection caused by the varicella-zoster virus. It is usually a mild disease for most people, although babies, those with compromised immune systems, and those taking steroids for other conditions are at risk for possibly serious complications.

Once contracted, symptoms begin to show in about two weeks and continue for another week to ten days. Fever, headache, and general malaise (a feeling of discomfort, illness, or uneasiness)

HEALTH

WELL-BEING

BEAUTY

HOME

develop first, followed by red bumps that become filled with fluid. These break and scab over. Hundreds of these itchy blisters form all over the body. This disease is highly contagious to those who have never had the virus before. It is spread mainly from touching the blisters of an infected person and through breathing in the virus suspended in air droplets. In otherwise healthy individuals, medical treatment is often not necessary. The infection is self-limiting and will clear on its own. Calamine lotion or oatmeal baths may help with itching, and nonaspirin medications can help reduce fever. Aspirin use in children with chicken pox has been associated with Reye's syndrome, a serious disease that affects the liver and brain. Vaccines are available and are 98 percent effective at preventing chicken pox.

In some countries, availability of the chicken pox vaccine or antiviral drugs is low, whether due to financial, religious, geographical, or other logistical factors. While honey can't be used to prevent chicken pox, it can be used to help the body heal faster. It is widely available and safe, a practical home remedy that people in most parts of the world can easily use. Honey will help reduce inflammation, pain, and itching and increase patient comfort. It has also been shown to have antiviral activity. Manuka and clover honeys were added to tissue cultures containing human cells infected with chicken pox; both types of honey showed significant antiviral activity against the varicella-zoster virus.[11]

For topical (on the skin) application, gently warm the honey and smooth it over the blisters in a thin layer. Leave on for about fifteen minutes and gently wipe off with a warm cloth. Repeat several times a day.

7. COLD SORES

Cold sores, or fever blisters, are herpes simplex viral (HSV-1) infections that affect the skin around the mouth. Fluid-filled sores develop in and around the lips, eventually breaking and leaking a clear liquid. A crust then forms. Cold sores tend to group in clusters and are red, swollen, and sore; these sores can be accompanied by fever and swollen neck glands. Some cold sores only last a few days, while others take weeks to go away.

The herpes simplex virus is contagious, and touching the area or sharing utensils, toothbrushes, or razors can spread the infection. The virus gets into the skin through any scratch or tiny cut, so if an outbreak is underway, don't kiss anyone goodnight or share a glass of wine! Once the virus is contracted, it will always be there. It is not always known why an outbreak occurs, but stress and a depressed immune system are thought to be triggers. Antiviral creams, ointments, or pills can reduce symptoms but usually only clear the sores one or two days quicker than without treatment.

Those few days, however, can be extremely important to people during an outbreak. The sores cause not only pain but also embarrassment for some. The initial tingling sensation associated with an impending outbreak can have a person running for medication or even hiding out until the cold sores have cleared up. One of the popular medical remedies to treat cold sores is acyclovir cream. This antiviral drug does not prevent contracting the virus causing cold sores, but it can help prevent actual sores and blisters from appearing.

HEALTH

WELL-BEING

BEAUTY

HOME

Many may be interested to know that honey is more effective than acyclovir in managing the symptoms of cold sores. A study investigated people with recurrent attacks and applied honey for one attack and acyclovir cream for another. Compared to acyclovir treatment, honey was better at reducing the duration of the symptoms by 35 percent, pain by 39 percent, occurrence of crusting by 28 percent, and average healing time by 43 percent. Two of the eight patients in the honey group had their symptoms completely disappear. This did not happen in the acyclovir treatment group.[12]

Dabbing honey on the affected area of the lips during the first sign of an outbreak and applying throughout the attack should resolve the lesions sooner.

8. CORONARY HEART DISEASE

When plaque builds up inside the arteries, coronary heart disease results. This plaque is comprised of cholesterol, fat, calcium, cellular waste products, and fibrin, a protein involved in blood clotting. Over time, the plaque builds up on the artery wall and hardens. The artery opening narrows and the flow of oxygen-rich blood to the body is reduced. Arteries to the heart, brain, arms, legs, kidneys, or pelvis may be involved.

If a piece of the plaque breaks off and is carried to another part of the body, it can get stuck in a smaller artery and cut off blood flow at that point. Sometimes blood clots form on the surface of plaque and block the artery entirely at the site of the plaque. If the blockage is to the heart, a heart attack will result. If it's to the head, a stroke occurs.

Coronary heart disease can begin in childhood but most often presents itself later in life. Smoking, a sedentary lifestyle, high blood pressure, poor diet, and genetics are all risk factors that can lead to its development. Changes in lifestyle and ongoing medical care are often required to minimize damage and manage this disease.

Studies show that in pretreatment with Sundarban honey, rats were protected from the destructive effects that heart attacks have on the body. Rats that received honey before induced heart attacks did not have significant increases in total cholesterol, low-density lipoprotein cholesterol, or triglycerides like the rats who did not receive honey. Their high-density lipoprotein cholesterol was not reduced, lipid peroxidase products were not increased, and anti-oxidant enzymes were not decreased. In fact, these levels were all near normal in the honey-treated group.[13]

It could be the phenolic compounds in honey that provide the protection to the heart and arteries, since taking it regularly is associated with a reduced risk of heart disease.[14] These phenolic compounds reduce blood clots and the tension in blood vessel walls, allowing for greater ease of blood flow. They also play a role in preventing the oxidation of low-density lipoprotein cholesterol, a key contributor to coronary heart disease.[15]

9. CROHN'S DISEASE

Crohn's disease is a chronic inflammatory bowel disease affecting sections of the lining of the digestive tract, particularly the deep tissue of the small bowel and beginning of the colon. Symptoms develop gradually and can flare up suddenly and disappear for

HEALTH

WELL-BEING

BEAUTY

HOME

periods of time. Many people with Crohn's suffer from stomach pain and cramps, diarrhea, poor appetite, rectal bleeding, fatigue, and fever.

While some people with Crohn's disease find it runs in their family, most discover no such genetic link. The cause is unknown, but viral or bacterial infections may trigger the immune system, setting off an abnormal response that tells the immune system to attack cells of the digestive tract. In severe cases, surgery is sometimes recommended for treatment, but most patients are treated with anti-inflammatory or immune-suppressing drugs to reduce inflammation or antibiotics to kill harmful intestinal bacteria.

This disease can be very debilitating and severely impact the quality of life of those afflicted. In some cases, medications don't completely reduce or prevent flare-ups. Alternative therapies need to be identified to assist with this. Diet can influence how our body reacts to genetic and environmental stresses and can induce pathways that allow disease to develop. Honey consumption was found to significantly decrease the risk of developing Crohn's disease. This became evident when dietary intake questionnaires given to newly diagnosed Crohn's patients and healthy subjects were analyzed. Whether it does so directly or influences other factors playing a role in its onset is still unknown.[16] Either way, consuming honey may provide some protection against developing this disease.

10. DIABETES

Diabetes is a disease that affects the way the body handles glucose, resulting in high levels of this sugar in the blood. There are three types of diabetes: type 1 diabetes, in which the pancreas produces little or no insulin; type 2 diabetes, in which the pancreas does produce insulin, but the body doesn't use it as well as it should; and gestational diabetes, a form of high blood sugar affecting pregnant women. Some people are genetically predisposed to diabetes, but being overweight is also a risk factor. Feelings of thirst, frequent urination, fatigue, tingling, numbness in the hands or feet, and blurry vision are all signs of diabetes. Managing diabetes involves exercising, improving diet, and monitoring blood glucose levels. For many, daily insulin injections are needed.

It may seem that honey, being a sweet substance, would not be good for diabetic patients; however, it does not have the same effects sugar has on the body—in particular, on glucose levels. Twelve weeks of honey consumption in patients with type 1 diabetes found that fasting serum glucose was significantly decreased. This is great news for those trying to keep their glucose at healthy levels. Furthermore, honey lowered total cholesterol, triglycerides, and low density lipoprotein levels. These are often elevated in diabetics and increase the risk of cardiovascular disease. Even subscapular skinfold thickness was lowered, indicating a reduction in body fat.[17]

Overweight and obese individuals are at greater risk of developing diabetes and having other metabolic abnormalities that may lead to diseases. Another study tested the effects in diabetic patients who inhaled a 60 percent honey spray. Honey significantly lowered blood glucose levels after thirty minutes. Fasting blood glucose levels taken three hours later were also reduced.[18]

Eating honey, especially in place of sugar, is beneficial to diabetics. We should take our cue from Ayurveda. It has long used honey in medicines for the treatment of diabetes.

11. DIABETIC FOoT uLCERS

One of the complications of diabetes is the development of ulcers (open sores) on the feet and lower legs. They are quite common in diabetic patients—up to 10 percent develop them.

When blood sugar levels are not well maintained or fluctuate regularly, nerve damage can result, most often in the legs and feet. These nerves are responsible for carrying pain sensation messages from the feet or legs to the brain. If not functioning properly, these messages aren't relayed, and damage to the skin may result. Another cause is a reduction in blood flow to the feet and legs because of narrowed arteries. This makes it difficult for skin to heal itself properly after injury and often results in an ulcer. Ulcers can take a long time to heal and be very uncomfortable. More serious ulcers may need amputation of the foot or limb.

Treatment must begin promptly to avoid skin and bone infections or gangrene. Because these ulcers heal slowly, the risk of infection is greater compared to other types of wounds. Usually, antiseptics like povidone-iodine are applied to the wounded skin, but honey is also a treatment that could be used. One study looked at the effects of both povidone-iodine and honey in dressings placed over diabetic foot ulcers. The average healing time was similar in both groups, indicating that honey is as effective as the povidone-iodine.[19]

Using a high-potency honey like manuka could be even more effective. Manuka honey–impregnated dressings were applied to patients with diabetic foot ulcers. A similar control population received conventional dressings. It took an average of thirty-one days to heal the ulcers in the manuka honey group compared to forty-three days in the conventional dressing group. The ulcers were also rapidly sterilized in 78 percent of the honey group during the first week. Only 36 percent of patients' ulcers were sterile in the control group.[20] Even nonhealing ulcers can be mended with topically applied raw honey. One case report described nonhealing, antibiotic-resistant ulcers fully healing within one year of honey-dressing use.[21]

12. FOoD POISONING

Escherichia coli (E. coli) is a bacterium that normally lives in the intestines of humans and animals. Many types of *E. coli* are harmless and are important to the health of the digestive tract. Several species, however, are pathogenic (cause disease) and can produce bloody diarrhea, urinary-tract infections, anemia, or kidney failure.

Contraction of *E. coli* can be made from contact with infected persons or animals or from consuming food or water containing the bacteria. *E. coli* can contaminate meat during processing, and if it is not cooked to 160 degrees Fahrenheit (71 degrees Celsius), it can survive and infect the consumer. Sometimes cows spread the bacteria to their milk as it passes their udders. If the milk is not pasteurized, the bacteria will continue to live and pose a threat. Even raw fruits and vegetables can have *E. coli* bacteria from contact with contaminated water or people. Three or four days after ingesting *E. coli*, food poisoning becomes evident as symptoms (nausea, vomiting, adnominal pain, cramps, fever, water or bloody diarrhea, or dehydration) develop. They usually subside on their own after about a week.

Salmonella bacteria can cause food poisoning too. They enter the system through processing and handling of contaminated poultry, beef, milk, eggs, and even vegetables. *Salmonella* is also found in some pets, ducklings, reptiles, hamsters, and other small rodents. Hand washing is recommended after handling these animals to prevent infection. If *Salmonella* poisoning does happen, it usually occurs within twelve to seventy-two hours after it enters the body. Diarrhea, stomach cramps, and fever develop and can last up to a week. They eventually subside without medication.

There is no way to know if produce contains *E. coli* or *Salmonella* bacteria because the food looks and smells normal. The best way to avoid infection is by prevention, so be sure to wash all produce before consuming and cook meats and other foods to their proper temperatures.

Despite our best efforts, sometimes these bacteria remain active in our food and can make us feel very sick. Consuming honey on a daily basis as a preventative to food poisoning may be enough to avoid getting sick or reduce the severity and duration of the illness. *E. coli* can be particularly difficult to eliminate because they readily form biofilms, which are slimy masses of bacteria that adhere to each other and other surfaces. They are highly resistant to anti-microbial agents, but honey has proven to be deadly to them. Low concentrations of honey have been able to significantly reduce bio-film formation of an *E. coli* bacterial strain that causes outbreaks of bloody diarrhea. When the biofilms were already formed, how-ever, this low concentration of honey had little effect in destroying them. It's important then, to ensure honey is taken as a preventa-tive to *E. coli* food poisoning.[22]

Honey also reduced the number of *Salmonella* bacteria that adhered to the outer layer of intestinal cells in a laboratory setting.[23] This indicates that in the body honey may be able to prevent *Salmonella* from thriving and multiplying in the intestines. Adding garlic to honey, specifically tazma honey (produced by stingless honeybees), significantly increases its potency against *Salmonella*.[24]

The type of honey can determine the extent of the antibiotic potential. Ziziphus honey, from the sacred tropical evergreen known as Christ's thorn jujube, effectively destroys both *E. coli* and *Salmonella*.[25] Ulmo 90 honey from the Patagonian rainforest has similar effectiveness as manuka honey against *E. coli*.[26]

Honey can be used as a natural alternative to antimicrobial drugs and may be used to prevent food poisoning or lessen the symptoms. A teaspoon of honey can be dissolved in a cup of warm water and sipped throughout the day. This can be repeated every four hours.

13. GANGRENE

Gangrene is a serious condition in which a lack of blood flow or severe bacterial infection causes body tissue to die. It most often affects the toes, feet, fingers, and hands and can result from injury, infection, or conditions that affect blood circulation, including diabetes and atherosclerosis.

Other parts of the body can be affected, such as the genitals and surrounding area. Gangrene in the genital area is called Fournier gangrene and is caused by multiple microbial invasions. It is a serious medical condition that can be recognized by sudden pain, rapidly followed by tissue swelling, which turns skin

HEALTH

WELL-BEING

BEAUTY

HOME

reddish-purple or bluish-gray. The tissue, or skin, starts to die and, as it decomposes, gives off a strong, foul smell. Treatment must be swift because the bacteria may pass into the bloodstream and the body may go into septic shock. This is life-threatening. Once gangrene begins, it cannot be reversed. The goal is to prevent further tissue damage. Doctors may perform surgery to remove the dead tissue and prevent the gangrene from spreading. Antibiotics are also prescribed.

The death rate for this infection is high, 20 to 30 percent on average, despite treatment with antibiotics and surgery. Any extra measure to fight the bacteria is welcome. Unprocessed honey dressings added to the treatment regime in patients with Fournier gangrene had better clinical and cosmetic results than patients who did not have honey applied to their infected skin.[27] This extra step could decrease the mortality rate for patients and increase their quality of life.

14. GASTRIC ULCERS

Ulcers are holes in the protective lining of the stomach, small intestine, and esophagus. Sores develop that may cause stomach pain, bloating, heartburn, nausea, and fatty-food intolerance. Infection with *Helicobacter pylori* is thought to be the main cause. Overuse of painkillers, smoking, stress, and heavy alcohol use are other contributing factors. If *H. pylori* bacteria are present, treatment involves a course of antibiotics to kill the bacteria. Medications to neutralize, block, or reduce the production of stomach acid are often prescribed. It is imperative that painkiller use, smoking, and alcohol use are greatly reduced or stopped.

Honey can be a great aid in the treatment of ulcers. A study conducted of patients testing positive for the *H. pylori* infection (using a urea breath test) were given a combination of approximately five teaspoons of honey and black cumin a day. After two weeks, the patients were again given a urea breath test. This time, 57 percent of participants had undetectable levels of *H. pylori*, indicating that the infection had cleared and the risk of gastric ulcers from these bacteria was eliminated.[28] In addition, the symptoms of indigestion were reduced.

Another study, this time in rats with acetic acid–induced gastric ulcers, found that treatment with manuka honey preserved proteins needed to secrete mucus and defend the stomach lining against acid damage. Honey's antioxidant and anti-inflammatory properties also provided protection and helped significantly lower the number of cells dying in the lining of the stomach.[29]

Taking a spoonful of honey daily or adding it to lukewarm teas or on toast can help heal gastric ulcers, whether from an overabundance of stomach acid or from a *H. pylori* bacterial infection.

15. GENITAL HERPES

Many people in the United States have genital herpes and don't know it. This is a viral infection, mainly from the herpes simplex virus type 2 (HSV-2), and less commonly from the herpes simplex virus type 1 (HSV-1). It is spread through sexual contact and is highly contagious.

Often, the infection displays little or no symptoms. If symptoms are present, they may include itching and pain in the genital area and sores that look like small red or white bumps that can rupture and ooze, eventually scabbing over. Repeated outbreaks are common, but symptoms are usually milder after the initial outbreak. There is no cure for genital herpes, though treatment with antiviral medications can help heal sores more quickly and lessen the frequency of recurrences. The treatment can also minimize the chance of passing the virus to others, which is particularly important since the virus can be transmitted in the presence or absence of visible sores.

Medications for genital herpes are only available through prescription. An alternative that is easily accessible and cost-effective is honey. Patients with recurrent attacks of genital herpes were treated with honey for one attack and acyclovir cream for another attack. (This drug is commonly used to treat herpes by blocking the DNA of the virus so that it cannot replicate.) Comparison of the treatments found that honey reduced the average length of the attack by 53 percent, pain by 50 percent, crusting by 49 percent, and healing time by 59 percent better than acyclovir. No side effects were observed with honey, while a few patients had localized itching where acyclovir cream was used.[30]

A thin layer of honey can be topically applied to the affected areas of the skin to speed healing and reduce pain.

16. GINGIVITIS

Gingiva means "gum"; when the part of the gum around the base of the teeth becomes diseased, the condition is referred to as "gingivitis." The gums tend to bleed easily, become puffy, and turn from pink to red. They begin to recede, and tooth decay sets in.

Gingivitis is caused when hardened plaque, called tartar, forms below and above the gum line. Tartar is full of bacteria, the same bacteria that begins the infection. Plaque is formed daily on the teeth, but it can easily be removed through daily brushing and flossing. If it is left to harden into tartar, however, it is much harder to eliminate. This disease is common and symptoms are often mild, so most people don't know they have it. Professional teeth cleaning is needed, followed by a good oral-hygiene routine at home.

Manuka honey has high antibacterial properties. For this reason, it was used to see how well it worked against gingivitis. Thirty volunteers were randomly assigned to chew or suck a manuka honey product with a UMF of 15 (high-quality manuka honey) or sugarless chewing gum for ten minutes a day after each meal. Three weeks later, significant reductions in plaque and bleeding were noted in the honey group, while no changes were observed in the gum group.[31] In orthodontic patients, honey greatly reduced bacterial counts of common plaque bacteria after chewing a honey product.[32]

Honey can be used to prevent cavities and gingivitis and may be especially useful for those with braces or who are prone to dental issues.

17. HIGH BLOOD PRESSURE

The force exerted against arterial walls as blood flows through them determines blood pressure. The pressure is measured in the arteries when the heart contracts (systolic) and when the heart is at rest (diastolic). It is determined by how much blood the heart

HEALTH

WELL-BEING

BEAUTY

HOME

pumps and the resistance it encounters as it flows through the arteries. Blood pressure sustained above 140/90 mm Hg (millimeters of mercury) is considered high and is called hypertension. This condition develops slowly over time, and many people have it without knowing. It can damage blood vessels and the heart. If left untreated, it can lead to heart attack and stroke.

Primary hypertension doesn't have any identifiable cause, although obesity, smoking, poor diet, lack of exercise, and high salt intake are some common risk factors. Secondary hypertension has an underlying cause and could result from drugs or certain medications, alcohol abuse, thyroid problems, or kidney issues. Hypertension responds well to changes in lifestyle. Exercising more, eating a nutrient-rich diet, reducing stress, and quitting smoking and alcohol consumption should bring blood pressure down.

There are also many drugs available to lower blood pressure, including thiazide diuretics to reduce blood volume, beta-blockers to slow down the heart rate, ACE inhibitors to block the action of some hormones that regulate blood pressure, and calcium channel blockers and renin inhibitors to widen the arteries. All these medications come with significant side effects like diarrhea, fatigue, dizziness, nausea, erectile dysfunction, and headaches.

Changes in lifestyle should be the first line of defense against high blood pressure. The use of natural foods to lower blood pressure can also assist in safely bringing down elevated blood pressure levels. This concept of food therapy is an essential part of traditional Chinese medicine. Practitioners of this healing system frequently prescribe honey as one of the best foods to lower blood pressure and recommend its consumption to self-manage this condition.[33] Ayurveda, another of the world's oldest medical systems, endorses the use of two teaspoons of honey mixed with one teaspoon of garlic juice, twice a day, to control blood pressure. Scientific studies in rats support this idea. One such study found that honey supplemented to hypertensive rats markedly reduced systolic blood pressure.[34] *Systolic hypertension is the most common type of high blood pressure in older people, so honey consumption may be advisable in this population.*

18. HIGH CHOLESTEROL

Cholesterol is a waxy, fat-like substance found in cells. It is necessary in order for the body to make vitamin D, hormones, and bile acids that help digest food. We produce cholesterol on our own, but we also get it in saturated fat and cholesterol-laden foods. It comes in two forms: HDL (the good) and LDL (the bad). High cholesterol is when there are high levels of cholesterol in the blood, both HDL and LDL. When there is too much LDL cholesterol in the body, however, it can build up in the arteries and increase the chances of getting coronary heart disease. Plaque, which contains cholesterol, builds up inside the arteries and cause partial or full blockage, leading to narrowing and hardening of the arteries. This can lead to a heart attack or stroke. Statins are drugs commonly prescribed to lower LDL cholesterol, but taking statins can cause intestinal problems and muscle inflammation.

Cholesterol levels respond well to changes in diet. Eating foods low in saturated fats and reducing intake of animal products, which are the contributors of cholesterol in the diet, will do wonders. Forty-eight type 2 diabetic patients were randomized to either receive honey or not receive honey for eight weeks. In the group of patients consuming honey, significant decreases in total cholesterol, LDL cholesterol, and triglycerides were found, while HDL cholesterol significantly increased.[35] Daily consumption of honey in children and teenagers with type 1 diabetes had the same effect on cholesterol levels. The protective effect of honey can be used in people of all ages to bring down high cholesterol levels.[36]

19. JOCK ITCH

Named for its tendency to develop in athletes, jock itch is a mildly contagious fungal infection of the groin area. It can develop when the fungus finds a warm, moist place to grow. The skin becomes reddened in the crease of the groin and often spreads outward to the inner thighs, genitals, and buttocks. The rash is characterized as itchy, dry, and scaly, with red pus-filled blisters that may ooze.

It tends to be much more common in men than women and in those that sweat heavily, have diabetes, have a weakened immune system, or wear tight underwear. It is spread from direct contact, so don't share towels or clothing with an infected person. Because this is the same fungus that causes athlete's foot, take care not to spread the fungus from the foot to the groin and vice versa. Keep both areas clean and dry to prevent the fungus from thriving. Antifungal ointments, lotions, or sprays can be used to clear mild infections in a few weeks. More severe infections or recurrent cases may require stronger prescription antifungal medication.

A honey solution of honey, olive oil, and beeswax can be spread over the infected area of the skin to help reduce redness, itch, pain, and scaling of the blisters. Over a four-week period, 78 percent of patients with jock itch had a positive clinical response when the solution was applied to their lesions three times a day. The fungal infection was completely eradicated in 71 percent of test subjects.[37]

HONEY JOCK ITCH SALVE

1 tablespoon honey
1 tablespoon olive oil
1 clove of garlic, quartered

1. Gently heat the olive oil on the stove and add the garlic. Warm over medium-low heat for about 10 minutes.
2. Remove from the stove and allow it to cool to a lukewarm temperature.
3. Discard the garlic, and mix in the honey until well incorporated.
4. Smooth this mixture evenly over the affected area of the skin. Leave on for 30 minutes.
5. Wash off. Reapply two to three times a day until the infection clears.

20. LEISHMANIA LESIONS

Leishmaniasis is a disease transmitted by sandflies infected with any of more than twenty species of *Leishmania* parasites. When these sandflies bite humans, they pass the parasite to the humans, causing infection. This disease affects millions of people and originates in over ninety countries worldwide. North Americans can become infected by traveling to or living in countries where the parasites are endemic.

The most common form is cutaneous leishmaniasis, which can develop into one or more skin sores. Symptoms often begin a few weeks to a few months after infection and begin as lumps on the skin. They develop into ulcers with a raised border. Some lesions are moist and will ooze pus, while others develop crusts or scabs over them. Generally, they are painless and resolve on their own, but this can take up to a year and cause ugly scarring. This can be troubling if the lesions are on the face, which is typical. Ulcers are susceptible to secondary infection and there are certain types that can also spread into the mucosal membranes (membranes that line the cavities in the body and cover the surfaces of internal organs) if not treated.

There are many treatments for cutaneous leishmaniasis lesions, but one that is effective and completely safe has not been found. It is for this reason that honey is of interest as a potential tonic to help heal these lesions. In lab settings, honey was found to have antiparasitic effects against three species of *Leishmania*.[38] The healing effects of honey on many types of ulcers is well documented to reduce ulcer size, pain, redness, and time to healing. In addition, honey is antimicrobial and impressively prevents secondary infections to wounds. High-quality raw honey with standardized antimicrobial activity would likely be the most efficacious honey to use in applying to *Leishmania* lesions.

21. MELANOMA

This is the least common but deadliest form of skin cancer. Melanoma occurs when a mutation in the DNA allows skin cells to grow out of control and form a cancerous mass. It develops most often on the sun-exposed areas of the skin, but it can also form in places protected from the sun's harmful ultraviolet (UV) radiation.

Other factors, such as a family history, skin type, number of moles, and a weakened immune system also increase the risk of developing melanoma. This cancer is characterized by large, brownish spots with dark speckles or dark lesions on the hands, feet, or mucous membranes (skin tissue that secretes mucus and lines many body cavities or organs). Moles may be melanoma if they change in color or size, bleed, or have irregular borders. Surgery, radiation, or topical medications are the conventional treatments for skin cancer.

Manuka honey has recently been studied for its effect on cancer cells. It was shown to be destructive to murine melanoma cells in a time- and dose-dependent manner, as it activates a metabolic cell pathway that leads to DNA fragmentation and cancer cell death. Used alone, manuka honey inhibited melanoma tumor growth in mice by 33 percent. In combination with paclitaxel, a chemotherapy drug, a 61 percent growth inhibition was observed.[39] This highlights honey's use alongside traditional cancer drugs to reduce dosage and lower the risk of side effects.

One of the compounds in honey, called chrysin, had previously been studied for its ability to decrease tumor size. Both chrysin and honey were tested for their effects on human melanoma cells. Both inhibited cell growth and replication.[40] Chrysin also appeared to be selective because it reduced the viability of melanoma cancer cells but did not affect healthy, normal cells.[41] This suggests that chrysin plays a major role in honey's anticancer activity and may be considered for further study in melanoma trials.

HEALTH

WELL-BEING

BEAUTY

HOME

22. MUCOSITIS

Cancer treatments of chemotherapy and radiation not only destroy rapidly dividing cancer cells but rapidly dividing epithelial cells as well. These cells line the gastrointestinal tract and include the lining of the mouth, throat, stomach, and intestines. When they are damaged, they become open to ulceration, and sores develop, a condition called mucositis. The most common place for these sores to develop is the mouth. Up to 40 percent of patients receiving radiation and chemotherapy develop mucositis. In addition to sores in the mouth, the gums can become swollen, red, and shiny. They can bleed or exude pus. Mucositis is very painful and can prevent swallowing in severe cases, leading to malnutrition. The severity of the condition is graded from 0 (no sores) to 4 (eating is impossible due to pain). Poor oral hygiene, smoking, drinking alcohol, chewing tobacco, and certain diseases increase the risk of developing mucositis.

No highly effective treatments of chemotherapy–induced oral mucositis have been found. Because honey is highly touted for its wound healing and anti-inflammatory properties, it has been investigated in recent years as a candidate to alleviate the pain and discomfort of mucosal sores. Patients with head and neck cancer were randomized to receive chemoradiation alone or chemoradiation and honey. The honey group consumed honey fifteen minutes before radiation, fifteen minutes after radiation, and before bed. After several weeks of treatment, patients in the honey treatment group significantly reduced their symptoms in grades 3 and 4 mucositis compared to the group who did not consume honey.[42]

Leukemia patients with grades 2 or 3 oral mucositis healed their lesions much faster applying honey than by just using benzocaine gel, a topical pain reliever.[43]

Honey use can also prevent the development of oral mucositis.[44] Betamethasone is another steroid used to treat inflammation and was less effective than honey when swallowed every three hours for one week. Interestingly, adding instant coffee to the honey was more effective than honey alone, although whether coffee has an additive or synergistic effect on honey's healing properties is undetermined.[45] Either way, it boosts the effectiveness of the treatment and can easily be mixed with honey.

These inexpensive home remedies can alleviate pain and improve oral function and quality of life in chemotherapy patients.

23. OUTER EAR INFECTION

Infections of the outer ear are very common and are caused by bacteria, although fungi are culprits too. Swimmers, those with narrow ear canals, and those with skin problems like eczema or psoriasis tend to be more affected. The warm, moist environment in the ear is the perfect breeding ground for bacteria or fungi that are commonly found in water or on the skin. They will readily invade the skin and multiply. The infection causes itching and redness, which can escalate to severe pain in and around the ear, discharge of pus, fever, and partial or complete blockage of the ear canal. To stop the infection, doctors commonly prescribe antibiotics, antifungals, or eardrops that contain both of these, and steroids. Taking over-the-counter pain medications such as ibuprofen is also recommended.

HEALTH

WELL-BEING

BEAUTY

HOME

Outer ear infections are very common and can be extremely painful if left untreated. Honey drops can be added to the infected ear to kill the bacteria and decrease itch, pain, and redness. In a recent study, patients with dermatological conditions leading to an infection of the outer ear were given medical-grade honey eardrops. They were applied daily in the affected ear for a period of two weeks. Patients were highly satisfied with the results and did not experience any negative side effects. Itch decreased, and over-all comfort increased.[46]

Dogs are also highly susceptible to outer ear infections. One milliliter of medical-grade honey was applied to the infected ears of dogs each day for up to three weeks. Seventy percent of dogs were completely cured within one to two weeks, with 90 percent being healed by the end of week three.[47] Medical-grade honey with standardized antibacterial activity can be used to restore health to the ear.

24. PROSTATE CANCER

This is cancer that occurs in a man's prostate, the small gland that produces seminal fluid to nourish and transport sperm. It can begin when some cells in the prostate mutate and begin to grow and divide rapidly. They live long after normal prostate cells die, and they come together to form tumors. These tumors can grow to invade nearby tissue, or some abnormal cells can break off and spread to other parts of the body. Some prostate cancers grow slowly and remain confined to the prostate. These often require minimal treatment and monitoring. Other types can be more aggressive and spread quickly. These need more invasive treatments and usually consist of surgery, chemotherapy, radiation, or hormone therapy. Advanced cases may cause difficulty urinating, slow urine stream, blood in the semen, erectile dysfunction, and bone or pelvic pain.

One of the compounds found in honey, chrysin, has both antioxidant and anticancer potential. Human prostate cancer cells were cultured with either chyrsin or honey for three days to determine their effect on the cancer cells. Both decreased cancer cell numbers in a dose- and time-dependent manner. Chrysin was observed to cause cell death, preventing further growth and multiplication of the prostate cancer cells.[48] Honey, especially with its component of chrysin, has promise as both a preventative and treatment of prostate cancer.

25. PSEUDoMONAS INFECTION

Pseudomonas bacteria are found in soil and water throughout the world. They thrive in moist areas like hot tubs, sinks, toilets, underchlorinated pools, and even outdated antiseptic solutions. Infections can include swimmer's ear, eye infections, wounds, urinary-tract infections, and pneumonia. Severe infections of the bloodstream, bones, joints, or heart valves can have severe consequences on health. Often, the use of medical devices increases the risk of infection. Many cases begin in hospitals. Those with weakened immune systems, diabetes, or cystic fibrosis also have an elevated risk. External infections are usually treated with oral antibiotics, while internal infections require IV administration.

HEALTH

WELL-BEING

BEAUTY

HOME

Chronic wound infections caused by *Pseudomonas* are difficult to treat because the bacteria have the ability to form biofilms, which are slimy matrices of the bacteria that cling to each other and to other surfaces. These tend to be very resistant to antimicrobial drugs. Medihoney, a wound dressing made from manuka honey, was proven to prevent biofilm formation and, at higher concentrations, inhibit the proliferation and viability of established biofilms.[49] Both manuka honey and a pasture honey were effective at inhibiting the growth of seventeen different strains of *Pseudomonas* isolated from skin burn wounds. Diluting the honeys tenfold did not diminish their antibacterial activity.[50]

Honey is effective because it works against this type of bacteria by crippling several of its processes and structures. It destabilizes the bacteria's cell wall; it deflagellates the bacteria so they cannot swim, adhere to tissue, and form biofilms;[51] and it limits the bacteria's ability to obtain iron from their host, which is needed for the infection to take hold.[52]

Altogether, honey is an effective agent in combating *Pseudomonas* and may help heal wounds faster or even prevent the infection from occurring.

26. RENAL/KIDNEY CANCER

Renal, or kidney, cancer is one of the ten most common cancers in both men and women. The kidneys are small, bean-shaped organs that lie behind the abdomen on both sides of the spine. Although we have two, only one is necessary to carry out its function of filtering waste products and excess water and salt out of the blood. The kidneys also help control blood pressure and red blood cell levels. Cancer in the kidneys begins when cells in the kidneys mutate and begin to divide out of control. The cells come together to form one or more tumors. The early stages of this disease rarely show any symptoms, but in the later stages, the patient may see blood in the urine, have back or side pain that doesn't go away, feel tired, or lose weight. Small tumors can be destroyed by freezing or heating the cancer cells, but often surgery is required to remove the tumor from the affected kidney or even the whole kidney, if necessary. Advanced cases may need drug therapy and radiation in addition to surgery.

Honey contains antioxidant compounds that are thought to have preventative effects against cancer. To investigate this premise in renal cancer, human renal cancer cells were treated with various concentrations of honey for three days. Honey decreased the ability of the cancer cells to survive by inducing the cells to program their own death. Higher concentrations of honey were more effective, as were longer exposure times.[53] Honey appears to be a promising candidate in treating renal cancer by preventing tumor growth.

27. RHEUMATOID ARTHRITIS

Rheumatoid arthritis is an autoimmune disorder in which the immune system mistakenly attacks its own body tissues. The lining of the joints becomes painfully swollen, and the condition can

HEALTH

WELL-BEING

BEAUTY

HOME

lead to bone erosion and joint deformity over time. Symptoms can spread to other nonjoint tissues of the body.

It's not known what causes this disease, but genetics combined with environmental triggers are suspected. This chronic disease is without a cure and is managed mostly through medications. Nonsteroidal anti-inflammatory drugs, steroids, or disease-modifying antirheumatic drugs can be prescribed to reduce pain, swelling, and joint damage. Possible side effects include digestive problems, liver and kidney damage, heart problems, thinning of bones, diabetes, weight gain, and severe lung infections.

Indian medical practice has long used Kalpaamruthaa, an herbal preparation, to treat arthritis. It consists of honey, marking nut, and Indian gooseberry. All three are known to have therapeutic compounds. In a study, three treatments were used to assess their anti-inflammatory activity and their effect on arthritis: the herbal preparation, marking nut, and the nonsteroidal anti-inflammatory drug diclofenac sodium. The herbal preparation that included honey was the most effective in reducing swelling and improving arthritis. It is believed that combining honey with marking nut and Indian gooseberry provides a mixture of phytochemicals that work with each other to improve arthritis.[54]

28. RINGWORM

Despite its name, worms do not actually cause this condition. Ringworm is a fungal infection of the outer layers of skin that is characterized by a red rash that forms a circle, or ring, on the surface of the skin with a clearer patch of skin in the middle. The fungus can affect any area of the body with one or many rings. It is contagious. Even touching bedding, towels, or surfaces that were in contact with the fungus can cause it to adhere to the skin and begin to multiply. Children are most susceptible. Initially, the rash is red, itchy, and flat. If it progresses, the skin can become inflamed with pus-filled blisters. Over-the-counter fungal creams can be used to get rid of the infection, but in severe cases, prescription antifungal medications may be needed.

An easy, at-home remedy that may prove highly effective is honey. Patients with clinically diagnosed ringworm were given a mixture of honey, beeswax, and olive oil to apply to the affected skin three times a day for up to four weeks. Seventy-five percent of the patients saw a reduction in redness, itch, pain, and scaling of their blisters. Upon clinical examination, complete eradication of the fungus was determined in 62 percent of the cases.[55] The same salve used for jock itch may also be used for ringworm.

HONEY RINGWORM SALVE

1 tablespoon honey
1 tablespoon olive oil
1 clove of garlic, quartered

1. Gently heat the olive oil on the stove, and add the garlic clove, sliced into quarters.
2. Heat over medium-low heat for about 10 minutes.
3. Remove the mixture from the stove, and allow it to cool to a lukewarm temperature.
4. Discard the garlic quarters and mix in the honey until well incorporated.

HEALTH
WELL-BEING
BEAUTY
HOME

5. Smooth this mixture evenly over the affected area of the skin. Leave on for 30 minutes.

6. Wash off. Reapply two to three times a day until the infection clears.

29. SEBORRHEIC DERMATITIS

Seborrheic dermatitis is a common skin condition that mainly affects the scalp but can also appear on oily areas of the body, like the sides of the nose, eyelids, and chest. It is thought to develop from an improper immune response or from *Malassezia furfur*, a fungi commonly found on the oil glands of the skin. The skin can become red and itchy with patches of flaky white or yellow scales on the body or skin flakes noticeable in the hair, eyebrows, beard, or mustache. The skin flakes are commonly referred to as dandruff. Mild cases are easy to treat with daily cleansing to reduce oil and skin-cell buildup. Other cases are more difficult and may need medicated shampoos to reduce inflammation and kill the microbes.

Recent studies have shown honey to be effective against *Malassezia*.[56] If applied to the affected areas of the skin, honey can reduce the symptoms of the infection and even eradicate the fungus, preventing recurrence. This was demonstrated in a study in patients with seborrheic dermatitis. One group gently rubbed a honey solution (9 parts honey, 1 part water) into their skin every other day for several minutes. They left the honey on for three hours before washing it off. The other group did not use honey. After one week, all the patients in the honey group saw vast improvements in scaling and itching. Within two weeks, skin lesions were healed. At the end of the six-month study, some patients even believed they had less hair loss. No patients relapsed in the honey group, but in the control group (no honey used) most of them had a return of their symptoms.[57]

30. STAPHYLOCOCCUS INFECTION

There are over thirty types of bacterial *Staphylococcus* (staph) infections, but most are caused by *Staphylococcus aureus* (*S. aureus*). These bacteria are responsible for skin infections, pneumonia, food poisoning, blood poisoning, and toxic shock syndrome. Staph skin infections are most common and are usually minor. They look like pimples, blisters, or boils. More severe infections, however, can show red, swollen rashes with pus or drainage.

Many people carry these bacteria on their skin or in their noses without any symptoms. The bacteria get into the skin through cuts or scrapes, so it is important to keep wounds clean and to wash hands regularly. If the bacteria invade the body and get into the bloodstream, infections can turn up in numerous organs and become life threatening. Treatment for minor staph infections is usually a course of antibiotics or drainage of infected areas. Severe infections require hospitalization. Many varieties of staph have become resistant to antibiotics. New treatments are needed to continue to fight these ubiquitous bacteria.

HEALTH

WELL-BEING

BEAUTY

HOME

Manuka honey is a strong inhibitor of *S. aureus* infections. In 108 patients with chronic venous leg ulcers, sixteen had methicillin-resistant *S. aureus*. These strains are resistant to all types of penicillin. After four weeks of treatment with manuka honey, 70 percent of the wounds no longer had methicillin-resistant *S. aureus*. In the group treated with hydrogel dressing, only 16 percent of methicillin-resistant *S. aureus* were destroyed.[58] Hydrogel dressings are commonly used in wound care to promote healing and prevent infection.

Fortunately, it's not just manuka honey that works against the staph bacteria; the Chilean honey, ulmo 90, proved to have even better antibacterial activity against resistant *S. aureus* strains.[59] Honey acts against *S. aureus* single cells and biofilms, slimy masses of cells that are very difficult to eradicate. Up to 82 percent of the susceptible strains of biofilms and up to 73 percent of the resistant strains of biofilms were wiped out by honey.[60]

Honey can speed healing by preventing or clearing *S. aureus* infections, whether they are susceptible or resistant bacterial strains.

31. SUN FuNGuS

This condition is caused by the fungus *Malassezia*, which commonly reside on the skin of most people with no problems; however, when it grows out of control and causes an infection, it affects the normal pigmentation of the skin, resulting in patches that are lighter or darker than normal. It can cause some mild itching and scaling and becomes more noticeable with sun exposure.

It is not known precisely why such infections begin, but hot and humid weather, oily skin, hormonal changes, or a compromised immune system are contributing factors. This condition is not contagious and is found mostly in teenagers and young adults. Oral or topical over-the-counter antifungal medications can be used to return the skin to normal, but severe infections will likely require different medications prescribed by doctors. Pigmentation should return to normal after several weeks or months, but beware that this infection may return and medications will be needed again.

An easy and inexpensive at-home remedy that can help exterminate the fungus and alleviate symptoms is honey. A mixture of honey, olive oil, and beeswax was applied to the skin of patients three times a day for up to four weeks. Eighty-six percent responded well to the treatment and had improvements in itching and scaling. Seventy-five percent of the patients were fully cured of the fungus and saw complete resolution of their infection.[61]

Honey, olive oil, and beeswax can be mixed in equal proportions and spread over the skin, but honey has been used alone as well. Its antifungal activity extends beyond the *Malassezia* species. Honey destroyed this fungus on the scalp of patients with seborrheic dermatitis (commonly known as dandruff) and prevented the fungal infection from recurring.[62]

32. TAPEWORMS

Tapeworms are intestinal parasites that infect animals, including humans. Eating contaminated food or water containing microscopic tapeworm eggs or larval cysts, or coming into contact with infested soil and touching your mouth, is a sure way to get tapeworms. If eggs are ingested, they develop into larvae in the intestines and then move to other tissues, usually the liver and lungs, and develop into cysts. They can grow up to fifty feet long and live more than twenty years.

Many people with intestinal infections don't have any symptoms. Others experience nausea, diarrhea, weakness, weight loss, and abdominal pain. If cysts have developed in other organs of the body, the person may develop a fever, cystic lumps, or allergic reactions. Seizures have even happened with severe infections. Once diagnosed, oral medications to kill adult tapeworms are prescribed. If cysts have formed, they may need to be drained or removed by surgery.

If tapeworms are suspected or diagnosed, add honey to the diet. Test tubes containing at least five hundred juvenile tapeworms had various concentrations of honey added to them for up to ten minutes. Concentrations of just 10 percent honey were able to kill all the parasites, with death first being observed after three minutes.[63]

Honey appears to be a strong antiparasitic substance and may be useful as a preventative to an established tapeworm infestation by destroying one or more stages of the tapeworm's life cycle.

33. TUBERCULOSIS

Tuberculosis is an infectious disease caused by the *Mycobacterium tuberculosis* bacteria. It is spread when an infected person releases microscopic droplets containing bacteria into the air through coughing, sneezing, laughing, spitting, or talking. If these droplets are inhaled, the bacteria find a new host.

As many as thirteen million people in the United States have the tuberculosis bacteria in its latent form. This means it is present in the body but is inactive and no symptoms are evident. This form is not contagious, but it can turn into active tuberculosis, so treatment at this stage is still necessary.

Active tuberculosis is contagious because the bacteria have engaged in multiplying and affect the lungs and sometimes other parts of the body. Symptoms of chronic coughing with or without blood, chest pain, fever, fatigue, and night sweats become evident. Tuberculosis is the top infectious killer worldwide and the leading cause of death in HIV positive people. Current treatment with antibiotics lasts six to nine months unless the strain is drug-resistant, in which case a combination of antibiotics are prescribed for up to thirty months. Many strains of tuberculosis bacteria are resistant to one or more of these drugs, and the fear of more bacteria attaining this ability makes the future of tuberculosis treatment uncertain.

Honey is well known for its antibacterial activities. Because it is readily available and inexpensive compared to prescription medications, it has been looked at as a possible antibacterial agent to help improve the health of patients with tuberculosis.

One such study looked at formulations of Immunoxel—a water-alcohol extract of herbs—mixed with either honey, sugar, or gelatin. Tuberculosis patients were randomly assigned to be given one of these Immunoxel formulations once a day, along with their regular tuberculosis drugs. After one month, all formulations were effective in reducing the bacterial count, indicating that they are good choices to treat tuberculosis. An important difference, however, was when Immunoxel was combined with honey: 100 percent of the patients tested negative for the bacteria in their sputum. In contrast, the sugar, gelatin, and placebo formulations were only 70 to 90 percent (sugar), 77 percent (gelatin), and 19 percent (placebo) effective.[64] When evaluated in the lab, *Mycobacteria* was destroyed by a 10 percent honey solution.[65]

Some honeys are stronger than others. A 3 percent Pakistani beri honey solution eradicated all multidrug-resistant tuberculosis strains tested.[66] The significant antibacterial activity of honey, particularly with resistant strains of *Mycobacteria*, make it useful in managing tuberculosis and lessening the severity of the disease. Daily consumption may also be suitable as a possible preventative.

34. ULCERATIVE COLITIS

Ulcerative colitis is an inflammatory bowel disease that causes long-lasting inflammation in the innermost lining of the large intestine. The symptoms can vary depending on where the inflammation is located in the large intestine and are usually mild to moderate with periods of remission. Some signs of ulcerative colitis are diarrhea with blood or pus, rectal bleeding, abdominal or rectal pain, an urgency or inability to defecate, fever, fatigue, and weight loss. Treatment options include anti-inflammatory drugs or immunosuppressants. Severe cases may need surgery to remove the colon and rectum.

Along with inflammation, a decrease in antioxidants is often noted in ulcerative colitis. Honey can not only reduce inflammation but also has antioxidants that can lower oxidative stress, paving the way for gut tissue healing. In rats with induced ulcerative colitis, the administration of honey decreased chemical markers indicative of oxidation and inflammation that lead to cell death.

Honey also plays a role in the regeneration of damaged tissue in the intestinal lining.[67] Fourteen days use of manuka honey in rats increased antioxidant status and protected against colonic damage when colitis was induced.[68] Combining manuka honey with sulfasalazine, an anti-inflammatory drug, had an additive effect and significantly reduced colonic inflammation and improved antioxidant levels compared to either treatment used alone.[69] In another study on rats with ulcerative colitis, honey proved to be as effective as prednisolone, a steroid used to treat many inflammatory diseases.[70]

Whether used alone or combined with medications, honey appears to be useful in relieving the symptoms of ulcerative colitis and improving the health of the intestines.

35. URINARY-TRACT INFECTION

Urinary-tract infections involve any part of the urinary tract and include the bladder, urethra, kidneys, and ureters. Infections of the bladder are most common. Bacteria in the stool, commonly *E. coli*, can adhere to the skin and make their way into the urethra. Once there, the bacteria move up into the bladder and begin to multiply.

Initially, symptoms are not evident, but as the infection progresses, urine output changes. Many report a frequent urge to urinate, burning urination, and urine that smells bad or is cloudy, red, or pink. Pain in the pelvis or abdomen is sometimes experienced, and nausea and/or vomiting can occur. Most urinary-tract infections are treated with a course of antibiotics. Sometimes if the

HEALTH

WELL-BEING

BEAUTY

HOME

pain or burning sensation is severe, doctors may prescribe pain relievers to numb the bladder and urethra.

As a preventative for urinary-tract infections or for use in the early stages of an infection, consume honey daily. Honey effectively eliminates *E. coli*, the bacteria most often responsible for urine and bladder infections. These bacteria are prolific and readily form biofilms, which are slimy masses of bacteria that adhere to each other and other surfaces. They can be particularly difficult to eliminate because they are highly resistant to antimicrobial agents. The good news is that low concentrations of honey have proven to significantly reduce *E. coli* biofilm formation.[71] Manuka honey (UMF15+) is particularly strong at reducing *E. coli* biofilm development and can inhibit the attachment of these biofilms to vinyl, such as on urinary catheters. Biofilms on these medical devices can often lead to urinary tract infections.[72]

Making a warm tea with added honey to sip throughout the day can help rid the body of the infectious bacteria and eliminate uncomfortable symptoms.

HONEY CINNAMON TEA

1 cup warm, filtered water
1 teaspoon raw honey
1/4 teaspoon cinnamon powder
1/4 lemon

1. Heat the water until just warm, no more than 95 degrees Fahrenheit (35 degrees Celsius).
2. Add the honey, and slowly stir until it melts.
3. Sprinkle in the cinnamon.
4. Squeeze in the juice from the lemon.

Put this tea in a thermal container, and sip continuously throughout the day. When this is gone, make another cup. Consume three cups each day.

HEALTH

WELL-BEING

BEAUTY

HOME

CHAPTER 2

SAFEGUARD WELL-BEING

HEALTH

WELL-BEING

BEAUTY

HOME

36. AEROBIC PERFORMANCE

Aerobic exercise improves fitness by increasing heart and breathing rates for a longer than a few minutes. Blood gets pumped around the body, delivering oxygen to the cells to keep the muscles working. Increasing fitness improves not only physical health but mental and emotional health as well. Regular aerobic exercise strengthens the heart, makes the muscles more efficient at consuming oxygen, and increases the number of mitochondria in the muscle cells. These increase endurance and more efficiently burn fat and carbohydrates. Running, walking, biking, and swimming are some examples of aerobic activity. Many of us have a goal to increase our fitness, and there are numerous products on the market that promise to do this by improving stamina or building muscle. Some of these may work, but they often have a long list of questionable ingredients.

Raw honey is made up mostly of simple carbohydrates and is the perfect fuel for runners and other aerobic performers. Glucose sugar molecules are absorbed quickly and will give an immediate burst of energy. The fructose sugar molecules are absorbed more slowly, releasing energy over a greater period of time. Honey also contains vitamins and minerals to help replenish dwindling stores and none of the preservatives, artificial colors, flavors, and sweeteners that many of the commercial energy drinks and gels contain. It is thought to perform as well as most commercial energy products when used as a sporting fuel. Prolonged exercise depletes glycogen stores and results in fatigue. Honey can be used post-workout to increase subsequent performance.

In a tested scenario, athletes ran for sixty minutes in a temperature of 31 degrees Celsius (about 88 degrees Fahrenheit). During a two-hour break, they were given either a honey drink or water. They then ran another twenty minutes. Those that drank honey ran significantly greater distances than those who only drank water.[73]

Whether it's for initial fueling, during exercise, or as a recovery after exercise, honey can fuel the body, restore energy, and banish fatigue.

37. ALCOHOL INTOXICATION

Alcohol includes all forms of ethanol and is found in wine, champagne, beer, vodka, rum, whiskey, gin, tequila, brandy, cognac, and vermouth. It increases the effects of GABA, a neurotransmitter that sends messages to the brain and nervous system and slows down signals. Consuming excessive alcohol slows signals too much and leads to physical and mental impairment. The severity of these effects depends on any health conditions, how frequently and how much the person drinks, the weight of the person, whether the individual is taking medications, or if food is in the stomach.

Twenty percent of alcohol is absorbed into the bloodstream directly from the stomach and 80 percent from the small intestine, where it is metabolized in the liver. After one drink, the person's skin may feel flushed, and the individual may feel less inhibited. As more and more alcohol is consumed, slurring of speech, lack of judgment, poor coordination, emotional instability, and memory loss may be evident. Eventually the person may become stuporous or even comatose. Death is possible if blood pressure drops too low, breathing ceases, or vomit blocks the airways. Sobering up takes time. Cold showers and caffeine have a temporary effect and should not be relied upon to remove the symptoms of alcohol consumption. Medications won't speed up the removal of alcohol from the body, but nonsteroidal anti-inflammatories can help with the pain of a hangover.

Taking honey while drinking can reduce alcohol's effects on the nervous system, which usually slow down processes and lead to impairment. A single dose of honey orally administered thirty minutes before mice were intoxicated with ethanol increased activity in the nervous system that controls the internal organs like the heart and stomach, and some of the muscles. These functions are normally slowed by alcohol. Honey consumed after intoxication was found to significantly decrease blood ethanol concentration.[74]

Honey contains fructose, a type of sugar that helps the body metabolize alcohol into harmless by-products. This can greatly reduce the effects of alcohol and have a large impact on mental and physical functions.

38. ANAL FISSURES

An anal fissure is a small tear in the tissue that lines the anus. The most common causes are straining to pass hard or large stools, chronic constipation, prolonged diarrhea, childbirth, and anal sex. The fissures can be painful, especially during and after a bowel movement. Bright red blood on the stool or on toilet tissue may be evident, and the area may burn and itch. Visible cracks in the skin or small lumps near the anus are other symptoms. If the fissures have been an issue for many weeks, swelling and scar tissue may be present.

Adding more fiber to your diet and ensuring adequate hydration will produce softer stools that will be easier to pass. Exercise can promote regular bowel movements that often do not require straining to evacuate. Topical anesthetic creams can relieve pain temporarily. Anal fissures that do not heal may require surgery to reduce spasms and pain.

Honey can be used topically to ease pain and reduce inflammation. The antimicrobial activity of honey can prevent a bacterial or fungal infection from establishing itself in the area, which usually increases discomfort and healing time and leads to complications. A spoon-sized amount of a honey, olive oil, and beeswax mixture was topically applied by patients to their anal fissures twice a day. Follow up was every week for a maximum of four weeks. Pain, bleeding, and itching were significantly reduced, and no side effects were noted.[75]

Honey can be applied on its own or mixed with olive oil or both olive oil and beeswax in equal proportions and applied to the fissures. Place a piece of gauze over the mixture to protect clothes and prevent it from being wiped away.

39. ANXIETY

Everyone feels anxiety at certain times. Before going on a job interview, stepping out on a first date, or moving to a new city, you may experience fear, worry, nervousness, panic, or uneasiness. These feelings usually subside after the event has passed. For some, these feelings don't resolve and are persistent and overwhelming. This is another level of anxiety and is classified as an anxiety disorder. There are different types, but they can all interfere with normal life and be so intense and disabling that the afflicted withdraw from society.

Anxiety is caused by changes in the part of the brain that regulates emotions. On a physiological level, the person may have shortness of breath, heart palpitations, nausea, muscle tension, and insomnia. Drugs can be used to reduce symptoms, counseling to address emotional issues, diet changes to improve overall body function, and relaxation techniques to self soothe.

Some people with anxiety require the help of doctors and counselors to assist them in dealing with psychological issues and physical symptoms, regardless of whether anxiety stems from normal fear and worry or from a diagnosed anxiety disorder. Consuming honey can help decrease anxiety stemming from a variety of sources, including toxins and hormonal changes. Rats fed either honey, sucrose (sugar), or a sugar-free diet for one year saw remarkable differences in their mental state. The honey-fed rats had significantly less anxiety throughout the year when compared to the other two groups.[76] In rats with lead-induced neurotoxicity, honey protected against an increase in anxiety levels. Memory, locomotion, and antioxidant activities were enhanced.[77]

It is believed that the antioxidants in honey are the key in preserving brain function and preventing anxiety. In postmenopausal women, taking honey each day could alleviate anxiety, a symptom felt by some women during this time of hormonal change. Tualang honey given to female rats who had their ovaries removed (to simulate the menopausal condition) significantly reduced anxiety-like behavior, compared to the rats who had not received honey but who also had their ovaries removed.[78]

Though still being studied, honey has already proved a great success and may be tried in place of antianxiety medications.

....

40. APHRODISIAC

The term "aphrodisiac" originated from the Greek name *Aphrodite*, the Greek goddess of love, and can be a food, drink, or drug that stimulates sexual desire or excitement. Over the centuries, plant and animal products have been used to increase sexual desire and, in turn, enhance sexual performance and pleasure. The natural aphrodisiac inherent in our makeup is pheromones, chemicals emitted by the body and whose scent subconsciously attracts others by triggering physiological and behavioral responses. These can be supplemented with foods and other agents to increase desire and attraction.

Honey has been considered an aphrodisiac for centuries. Hippocrates, known as the father of medicine for his contributions in medicine, recommended honey for sexual vigor. Avicenna, the famous Islamic scientist who made significant and long-lasting contributions to medical science, is said to have advocated a mixture of honey and ginger as a sexual stimulant. He also favored it to cure impotence, or the inability in a man to reach an erection. Honey is supposed to increase nitric oxide levels in the body, which help muscles relax and blood vessels dilate. Blood flow then increases and can result in firmer, longer-lasting erections in men and more intense orgasms in both men and women.

41. BAD BREATH

No one wants bad breath, but everyone gets it now and then. Some foods, like onions and garlic, are common culprits for bad breath, and their strong odors linger until the food has been digested. Poor dental hygiene is another source of bad breath. Food particles that remain in the mouth become food for bacteria, which grow and thrive, emitting foul-smelling toxins into the mouth. Yeast infections, cavities, smoking, dry mouth, and some diseases are other causes.

Using mouthwash as part of an oral hygiene routine is optional, but many choose to include it. Most mouthwashes are antiseptic and are used to decrease the microbes in the mouth to prevent cavities, gingivitis, and bad breath. Others are advertised as reducing inflammation, pain, or dry mouth caused by infection or disease. About twenty milliliters of mouthwash is gargled for thirty seconds or more before spitting out.

It may seem counterintuitive to use honey as a mouthwash since it has a lot of sugar. We all know sugar is bad for teeth, as it feeds the bacteria in the mouth and leads to cavities if proper care is not taken. But honey also contains many antibacterial compounds and may be used to destroy the bacteria in the mouth. Without the bacteria present, the sugars are useless as fuel for them to grow and thrive. Manuka honey, in particular, has high levels of antibacterial compounds and may be more effective than some honeys with lower concentrations. Other honeys, however, contain hydrogen peroxide, and this is also antimicrobial. Even the low pH of honey works toward removing bacteria by creating an acidic environment that inhibits some bacterial growth.

HONEY MOUTHWASH

1 cup water
1 teaspoon honey
1/4 teaspoon cinnamon powder

1. Heat the water to less than 95 degrees Fahrenheit (35 degrees Celsius).
2. Stir in the honey until it melts, and add the cinnamon. Mix.
3. Gargle with this mouthwash morning and evening to fight bad breath.

42. BURNS

A burn causes damage to the skin and possibly underlying tissues and results from sunlight, heat, chemicals, electricity, or radiation. There are three types of burns. First-degree burns affect the outer layer of skin and cause minor inflammation, redness, and pain. Second-degree burns damage the outer layer of skin and the layer underneath. They are characterized by blisters, redness, and pain. Third-degree burns are the most serious and damage the deepest layer of skin tissue. They have a white, leathery appearance. Treatment for minor burns includes cleaning the wound, applying antibiotic cream, and taking pain medication. More severe burns should be treated by a medical professional.

First- and second-degree burns can use honey dressing to prevent infection, reduce inflammation, and allow the body to heal damaged skin tissue. It has shown to be more effective than commonly used commercial antibiotic dressings. Silver sulfadiazine is a topical antibiotic cream used to prevent and treat infections in burn tissue. It may cause pain, itching, burning, or upset stomach. Pregnant and breastfeeding women should not use it because it may possibly harm the baby. Honey is safe, however, and has been shown to be more effective than silver sulfadiazine.

Patients who received honey on one of their second-degree burns and silver sulfadiazine on another found that honey-treated burns healed much faster.[79] Honey showed satisfactory tissue growth over the wounded skin in 100 percent of patients after twenty-one days, while silver sulfadiazine only showed these results in 84 percent of patients. Honey was also better at reducing inflammation and infection,[80] relieving pain, and reducing the formation of scars.[81]

43. CANKERS

Canker sores are shallow ulcers that develop on the tongue or inside of the lip or cheek. They are round or oval with a red border and yellow or white center. A person may be afflicted with one or many at a time. Cankers can make it hard to eat and talk because they are very painful. The exact cause of cankers is unknown, but several contributing factors common among regular sufferers are stress, hormonal changes, food allergies, acidic food, irritation from braces, biting of the cheek, and nutrient deficiencies. While most minor cankers heal by themselves within several weeks, larger sores can take up to six weeks and can scar the tissue.

There is no treatment that will cure cankers. The best that can be hoped for is to prevent infection and manage pain while reducing the duration of the ulcer. Honey was tried as a topical treatment for cankers and compared to a topical corticosteroid (anti-inflammatory and immune-suppressing drug) and benzocaine (numbing medication) in the management of this condition. Patients were randomly allocated to receive one of the three treatments, which they applied four times a day for five days. Honey significantly reduced ulcer size, duration of pain, and redness of the skin compared to the other two treatments.[82]

44. CATARACTS

The most common cause of vision loss in people over forty is cataracts, which develop when the natural lens of the eye clouds over. The process can be gradual and happen with aging, or it can be a complication of certain medications or diseases, such as diabetes.

In the latter cases, the lens is often affected more rapidly. Proteins in the lens begin to break down and clump together, causing the cloudiness. Light entering the eye scatters, rather than focusing on the retina. The resulting symptoms include blurred vision, double vision, dulled colors, impaired night vision, and sensitivity to light. Having cataracts is like looking through fog or a dirty windshield. If vision is only minimally impaired, new eyeglasses may be all that is needed. If, however, diminished vision is impacting daily life, cataract surgery may be required. This is a simple, painless procedure that replaces the cloudy lens with an artificial, clear one. Most of those undergoing this surgery regain all or most of their vision.

Oxidative damage to the lens is one possible cause to explain the development of cataracts. Rat lens cells cultured in a high glucose medium significantly increased their oxidative stress and the cells began to die. When treated with propolis, a constituent of honey, oxidative stress was reduced and more cells survived. Oral administration of propolis also inhibited the onset of cataracts in 15 percent of at-risk rats and slowed the disease progression in 25 percent.[83]

Complications of cataract surgery can also be relieved by honey. Sometimes the interior of the eye can become inflamed, which can be serious; precautions are therefore needed. Often, topical antibiotics are used, but pathogens in the eye are becoming immune to them. A 25 percent honey solution was compared to a common antibiotic in preventing inflammation of the eye following cataract surgery. Eye drops of one or the other solution were administered both before and after surgery. Both greatly reduced the bacteria in the eyes to a similar extent.[84] This means honey is as effective as prescription antibiotics and can be used to help deter bacterial infections and surgical complications, as well as reduce the risk of developing cataracts and perhaps even slowing development. In the latter case, consuming pure propolis (also called "bee glue") may be better than honey to ensure effective concentrations are consumed.

45. COGNITIVE FUNCTION

The attainment and processing of knowledge is a direct function of cognition-mental processes that include perception, memory, reasoning, judgment, attention, and language. Each person is unique; how one sees and reacts to the world differs from how another does. Genetics accounts for the majority of cognitive variation seen in the general population. Environmental factors and physiological processes make up the rest. Chemical imbalances and changes in metabolic pathways can bring a noticeable change in cognition over time. Some of these processes can be triggered with age, dietary deficiencies, or exogenous chemical or pathogen exposure. Memory and thinking skills can become impaired.

Declining mental capacity can be distressing for the affected person and their loved ones. Getting enough sleep, exercise, and social stimulation can help, as can brain-training games. Dietary components can have an impact on cognitive ability too. Honey has been shown to counteract the memory-lowering effects of stress that can influence cognitive ability. Tualang honey orally fed to stress-induced rats once a day protected memory functions from declining, an outcome not seen in the honey-deprived rats. Honey also had an antidepressant-like effect on the rats.[85]

Depression affects thinking, concentration, decision-making, and other mental abilities. Taking honey every day may help provide essential nutrients to resist this decline.

46. CORNEAL SWELLING, POSTOPERATIVE

The cornea is the transparent tissue lying over the colored part of the eye. It focuses rays of light as they enter the eye and is integral in achieving sharp vision. The inner lining of the cornea contains endothelial cells, which constantly pump fluid out of the cornea. This keeps the cornea clear. If these cells are damaged, fluid fills the cornea, resulting in swelling, clouding of vision, and discomfort.

Corneal swelling can also be a complication of cataract surgery, despite improvements in surgical techniques and lens design. The natural lens of the eye that has developed a cataract is removed and an artificial lens implanted so that vision can be restored. During this process, some of the corneal endothelial cells are damaged. This condition may be temporary. The endothelial cells may restore their function and symptoms will disappear. It could also be permanent and may require surgery to fix.

Conventional topical therapies include corticosteroids (cortisone-like medications used to provide relief), drugs to lower fluid production, sodium chloride, and artificial tears. Sometimes these aren't enough to reduce corneal swelling, and additional measures are needed. In a recent study, two to three daily applications of antibacterial manuka honey eye drops were added to the eye-care routines of patients with persistent corneal swelling following ocular surgeries. After first putting in the drops, a temporary reduction in corneal swelling was observed and lasted for several hours. Habitual use of the drops improved vision and reduced damage to the epithelial cells of the cornea. Central corneal thickness also decreased,[86] meaning the health of the epithelial cells of the cornea improved. While further study would be helpful, it is clear the manuka honey eye drops improved eye health relating to corneal swelling.

47. COUGHS

Coughing is the body's reaction to irritated airways or a reflex action to remove mucus and foreign material from the lungs and upper airways. Smoke, dust, allergies, asthma, some medicines, bronchospasms, or an inhaled object cause dry coughs. Wet coughs result when mucus drains down the back of the throat from the sinuses or comes up the airways from the lungs. Infections, viruses, lung disease, postnasal drip, and smoking can cause mucus-induced wet coughs. People commonly buy expectorant medications (cough medicines that break up congestion) and suppressants (cough medicines that try to stop the cough reflex). These medications can become addictive and cause dizziness, drowsiness, nausea, and vomiting—even at recommended dosages.

Coughs can keep us up at night, affect daily activities, and cause pain in the throat and chest from irritated tissue and overexerted muscles. It is particularly distressing to see our children suffering from persistent cough, and many parents are looking for natural and safe solutions to help. Honey taken before bedtime can significantly improve nighttime cough and allow for restful sleep. Children with coughs and upper respiratory-tract infections who received a single dose of honey thirty minutes before bedtime reduced the severity and frequency of their coughs. Parent and child sleep quality was better.[87] When children were given either honey or dextromethorphan (cough medicine), both produced similar results. Parents did, however, rate honey more favorably than dextromethorphan for symptomatic relief.[88]

Another study found honey to be more effective than the cold medicine diphenhydramine.[89] In adults with persistent cough due to respiratory infection, one week of consuming a honey and coffee drink significantly reduced cough frequency and was better than prednisolone, a steroid used to treat chronic illnesses related to inflammation.[90] A simple honey mixture can help relieve the symptoms of a cough.

HONEY COUGH SYRUP

1/4 cup raw honey
1/4 cup water
2 tablespoons fresh lemon juice
1/2 teaspoon ground ginger

1. Combine all the ingredients in a clean jar.
2. Shake vigorously until thoroughly mixed.
3. Children can take ½ to 1 teaspoon and adults 1 tablespoon every few (3–4) hours.

48. DEPRESSION

Depression is a mood disorder that causes a deep sadness and a loss of interest in activities. It affects how a person feels, thinks, and behaves and can cause not just emotional problems but physical problems as well. Clinical depression may occur once in a person's lifetime or reoccur multiple times. This feeling of sadness and loss can cause insomnia, loss of appetite, poor concentration, fatigue, suicidal thoughts, and physical symptoms like backaches and headaches. Changes in the body's hormone levels may cause or trigger depression. Modifications of the way brain chemicals work and the effect it has on maintaining stable moods is thought to play a major role. Psychological counseling and antidepressant medications are often prescribed. Antidepressants can cause a wide range of side effects, including nausea, insomnia, blurred vision, weight gain, fatigue, and sexual dysfunction.

Diet can influence behavior, and the right foods or combination of nutrients may benefit conditions like depression. Tualang honey is one such food that may elevate mood. When rats were subjected to noise stress, those administered tualang honey were protected from experiencing depressive-like behavior compared to the rats that did not receive honey.[91]

One of the components found in honey that acts as an antidepressant is chrysin. Its antidepressant quality was demonstrated in a study in which mice were induced into a depressive state by having a part of their forebrain removed. This caused changes in the hippocampus, the thought center of the brain that controls emotion. When chrysin was administered to these mice over a fourteen-day period, the depression and changes in behavior were lessened. It performed similarly to fluoxetine, an antidepressant drug.[92]

No matter what the chemical compounds are or their mode of action, consuming honey may be beneficial in place of or alongside other treatments for depression.

49. DIAPER RASH

Diaper rash is a common condition in infants that causes the baby's bottom to become very sore, red, irritated, and tender. It is sometimes caused by the repeated rubbing of a soiled diaper against the baby's delicate skin. Diapers should be changed immediately after each bowel movement to avoid this. Allergens in baby wipes, lotions, and detergents may aggravate sensitive skin. If a diaper rash is suspected from any of these, each needs to be investigated and ruled out or selected as a possible contributor. Finally, diaper rash may be caused by a fungal or bacterial infection. The leak-proof nature of diapers keep baby's bottom warm and moist, which, combined with a change in pH from urine, creates a perfect environment for microbes to grow. *Candida albicans* is one of the main culprits causing diaper rash.

Make sure to frequently change diapers. Cleanse baby's bottom with mild soap and water and dry the area completely. Creams and ointments can be applied to the skin to create a moisture barrier to prevent future rashes. Within a few days, the rash should clear.

A safe and well-tolerated solution to improve diaper rash is honey. When honey was mixed with olive oil and beeswax and applied four times a day to the bottoms of babies with moderate to severe diaper rash, significant improvements in the rashes were observed after seven days. Even rashes caused by *Candida* can be improved by honey, which reduces the need for medicated ointments. Four of the babies' diaper rashes were from *Candida*. After seven days of honey treatment, two of the babies were cleared of the infection.[93]

DIAPER RASH OINTMENT

1/4 cup raw honey
1/4 cup olive oil
1/4 cup beeswax

1. Mix the three ingredients in a glass jar, and gently melt them in a pan of water on the stove over medium-low heat. Stir until the ingredients are well combined.
2. Remove from the heat, and allow the mixture to begin to cool. As it cools, the mixture may separate, so be sure to continue stirring until it has cooled to room temperature.

50. DIARRHEA

The term "diarrhea" describes loose, watery stools. It is a very common condition and usually lasts a few days, although prolonged diarrhea can indicate a medical condition like irritable bowel syndrome.

Stomach cramps and pain, bloating, fever, nausea, and vomiting often accompany diarrhea. It occurs when the stool moves too quickly through the colon, so the colon doesn't have time to absorb enough liquid from it. The main culprits for causing diarrhea are viruses, bacteria, and parasites. Food intolerance and many medications can also cause diarrhea in susceptible people. If diarrhea persists for more than a few days, doctors may prescribe antibiotics if the cause is bacterial or parasitic.

Increased resistance to antibiotics is a major problem in treating infectious bacterial diseases. Alternative therapies are needed to use instead of, or in combination with, current treatments for relief in resistant cases. Honey is an easily accessible and appetizing food that can effectively reduce the frequency of diarrhea and other symptoms like vomiting. When honey was added to a rehydrating solution and orally administered to children who were suffering from flu-induced diarrhea, they recovered more quickly compared to the children who received the rehydrating solution without honey.[94]

The antimicrobial and anti-inflammatory activity of honey may be responsible for quickly destroying the viral infection and reducing inflamed intestinal tissue, allowing for normal bowel function to return.

HEALTH

WELL-BEING

BEAUTY

HOME

51. DRY EYES

Tears are needed to ensure the health and comfort of our eyes. There are three layers to tears: an outer oily layer to keep tears from drying up too quickly, a watery middle layer to clean the eye by washing away particles and grit, and a mucus inner layer to help spread the watery layer over the eye and keep it moist. If production of one or more of these layers is diminished, dry eye can result.

Dry eye is a very common condition that affects millions of Americans and is more prevalent in women than men. Not only is it uncomfortable, it is downright irritating. The eyes can burn, itch, ache, or feel heavy and tired. They may be red and inflamed or sensitive to light. Wearing contacts can become painful. The overproduction of mucus or water may result as the eye's way of overcompensating, but this doesn't correct the underlying dry eye condition. The use of artificial tears can be helpful. If these drops are used frequently, be sure to purchase preservative-free brands so the chemicals in them don't irritate your eyes. Another option is to have an ophthalmologist insert a tiny device into the tear duct to block drainage and increase the eye's surface moisture.

A major cause of dry eye is wearing contact lenses. Honey eye drops can be used to alleviate the symptoms of dry eye and provide lasting relief. Contact-lens wearers suffering from dry eye found that adding honey eye drops twice a day for two weeks significantly improved their tear quantity and quality. Tears in dry eyes have less water and more salt than normal tears. The increase in salt concentration causes inflammation in the eye. Honey drops reduced inflammation of the eye caused by the condition. The more severe the symptoms, the better the drops worked.[95]

Dry eye can also cause an increase in the number of bacteria on the surface of the eye and on the eyelids, which increases the risk for chronic eye diseases. Ophthalmic honey applied to the inner lining of the lower eyelids significantly reduces the amount of bacteria present, almost to levels of people not suffering from dry eyes.[96] Check with your doctor before using honey eye drops, and make sure the honey used is medical grade.

52. ECZEMA

This is a group of medical conditions that cause the skin to become itchy and inflamed. It is often accompanied by asthma or hay fever and is common in infants, affecting up to 20 percent, although most outgrow eczema by their tenth birthday. About 3 percent of children and adults who experience it do so on and off throughout their lives.

During a flare-up, the skin is itchy, thickened, dry, and scaly. The skin may be red or brown, and pigmentation could be affected. There are many triggers that cause flare-ups, including scratching, hot showers, stress, clothing, or allergens. Nearly all people with eczema have *Staphylococcus aureus* bacteria on the skin, which multiple rapidly if they penetrate the surface. If this happens, symptoms worsen. Creams and oral drugs to control itching and inflammation can help manage symptoms, and antibiotics can help clear up an infection.

While corticosteroids (cortisone-like medications used to provide relief) are often effective in reducing redness, itching, and swelling associated with eczema, they may also aggravate these symptoms. Some users may also experience skin-color changes, acne, bruising, or the development of red or white bumps on the skin. Honey can be used instead to reduce skin redness, scaling, skin thickening, and itching. When applied to the skin in a mixture with equal amounts of olive oil and beeswax, 80 percent of patients showed improvement in their symptoms within two weeks.

Honey can also be used to replace a portion of the topical corticosteroid dosage when treating eczema.[97] Doing so reduces the risk of side effects without sacrificing potency of the treatment. If the skin is infected with *Staphylococcus aureus*, honey will also help treat this. It can destroy the bacteria, even when it's multidrug resistant[98] or in biofilm form.[99]

53. FEVER

Fever is a temporary increase in the body's temperature. It is not an illness but is a sign that something unusual is happening in the body. Mild fevers should be left untreated to allow the immune system to take care of the cause. Higher fevers are of more concern and require some intervention.

Sweating, chills, fatigue, muscle weakness, and headache may accompany fevers. They are generally caused by viruses, bacteria, some medications, sunburn, inflammatory conditions, and malignant tumors. Over-the-counter medications such as aspirin, acetaminophen, and prescribed antibacterial drugs are effective in reducing fever, but all come with risks. Aspirin can cause stomach pain, unusual bleeding, and weakness; overuse of acetaminophen can cause kidney and liver damage; antibiotics destroy good intestinal bacteria, causing digestive upset.

Honey is widely used in folk medicine to treat fever. A few ideas are to eat it straight out of the jar, combined with lemon and water in a tea, or mixed with cinnamon and spread on bread. A recent study found that daily consumption of honey and tahini (a condiment made from toasted sesame seeds) in acute myeloid leukemia patients reduced the duration and severity of fever. Fever is a common complication experienced by many of these patients due to a weakened immune system.[100]

Honey has antioxidants that counteract oxidative damage in the body, protecting immune cells from destruction and reducing its workload. The body can then focus on immediate concerns, like fighting the cause of the fever.

54. FLU

Seasonal flu is a respiratory illness caused by influenza A and B viruses. The viruses are contagious, and a person can become infected by touching a surface contaminated with the virus and transferring it to the mouth or nose. When this happens, the virus then nestles into the mucosal lining and begins to replicate. Contaminated people who cough or sneeze cause the virus to become airborne. Simply breathing in this air can begin an infection. Symptoms can be mild or severe and, in certain cases, be fatal. Symptoms include a fever, sore throat, runny or stuffy nose, cough, fatigue, muscle aches, and headaches. At its onset (within the first forty-eight hours of making its appearance), antiviral drugs can be taken to shorten the duration of the illness by one or two days and lessen the severity of symptoms.

Each year many people opt to get a flu vaccine to prevent seasonal influenza. This is not a guarantee that you won't get sick, however. If you do get sick and don't want to take antiviral drugs because of the possible side effects (including nausea, vomiting, diarrhea, and headaches), take honey to reduce symptoms and the duration of the illness. Manuka honey was shown to inhibit the replication of the influenza virus,[101] which limits its potency and shortens the period of sickness. When taken with two anti-influenza virus drugs, honey greatly reduced the amount of drugs needed for them to be effective.[102] Several teaspoons of honey can be consumed daily throughout flu season, either eaten straight off the spoon or in warm water with lemon, tea, or coffee (no hotter than 95 degrees Fahrenheit [35 degrees Celsius]).

55. HEARTBURN

Heartburn is also known as acid reflux. It occurs when acid splashes up into the esophagus from the stomach and causes a burning pain in the chest. Those who suffer from heartburn will notice that it is often worse after eating and at night. The acid travels more easily up the esophagus when the individual is bending over or lying down. Over-the-counter medications can be taken to reduce or neutralize the stomach acid, but these can sometimes cause nausea, constipation, diarrhea, headache, and abdominal pain—side effects that seem worse than the heartburn itself.

Taking a spoonful of honey soothes the throat and coats the esophagus, protecting it for a time from splashes of stomach acid and providing relief from the burning sensation. It may also reduce inflammation, which will ease pain.

Heartburn is associated with free-radical damage (caused by highly reactive molecules that can set off a chain reaction in a cell and destroy it) in the lining of the digestive tract. Because honey has antioxidants, it can protect against this damage by inhibiting the activity of free radicals. Honey also restores glutathione levels, an antioxidant that prevents cell damage. Glutathione is known to be lower in people suffering from heartburn. Try taking a teaspoon of raw honey after each meal and before bed.

56. HEMORRHOIDS

Hemorrhoids are swollen veins in the rectum and anus. The walls of the veins can stretch and cause the blood vessels to bulge. Internal hemorrhoids are inside the rectum and can bleed into the stool. This area has few pain receptors, so hemorrhoids here generally do not hurt. External hemorrhoids are located on the anus, where there are more pain-sensing nerves. These can be quite sore, especially during a bowel movement. They develop from a buildup of pressure in the lower rectum that can affect the flow of blood and cause the veins to swell. Straining during a bowel movement, pregnancy, or obesity can cause them. Hemorrhoids are extremely common and can explain bleeding, itching, pain, and inflammation. Topical creams or suppositories (a specially designed object that is inserted into the rectum or vagina to administer medicine), cold packs, and oral pain relievers can help subside symptoms.

Honey is anti-inflammatory and can reduce the swelling of hemorrhoids, along with redness, pain, and itch. When mixed in equal parts with olive oil and beeswax, it was found to do just that. Patients with first- to third-degree hemorrhoids applied a spoonful of this mixture to their affected areas twice a day for a maximum of four weeks. Bleeding was significantly reduced and itching relieved. No side effects were reported.[103] Once applied, place a square of gauze over the honey mixture to protect clothing and keep it from being wiped away.

57. HICCUPS

Hiccups are involuntary reflex contractions of the diaphragm, the muscle separating the chest from the abdomen. A quarter of a second after the diaphragm contracts, the vocal cords snap shut and cause the characteristic "hic" sound for which the condition is named. A single hiccup or a series of hiccups may start suddenly and often subside on their own within a few minutes. Excitement or stress, laughing, coughing, swallowing too much air, and some medical conditions like acid reflux or diabetes can trigger them. If hiccups persist for longer than two days, several medications can be prescribed that relax muscles, prevent spasms, or reduce acid reflux.

Hiccups can be incredibly annoying and disruptive. Everyone has an opinion on how to get rid of them, but there is no consensus on what actually works. Honey is the go-to remedy that many swear by. Mix a teaspoon of honey with two tablespoons of warm water, and stir until the honey melts. Slowly sip the solution, allowing the liquid to remain at the back of the throat for a second or two before swallowing. The honey supposedly stimulates the vagus nerve—part of the hiccup reflex control center. Signals to the vocal cords are then blocked, and normal function is returned.

58. INFERTILITY

The desire to have a baby strikes most people at some time during their lives. Many take for granted that they will be able to conceive a child, but that is not always the case. Approximately 15 percent of couples who have had unprotected regular sexual intercourse are unable to get pregnant after twelve months of trying or are unable to carry the pregnancy to full term.

A woman's fertility can be affected by irregular menstrual periods, a history of pelvic infections, uterine fibroids, endometrial polyps, or low egg numbers due to advanced maternal age. Men may have low sperm count, low sperm motility, or abnormal sperm shape. All these factors increase the risk of infertility. Medications are available to women to activate ovulation and egg development. If the man's sperm is the issue, intrauterine insemination is a possibility. The sperm are placed directly into the woman's uterine cavity to put them closer to the ovulated egg and increase the changes of insemination. In vitro fertilization is also used. The eggs are collected from the woman and fertilized with sperm outside of the body. The embryos are transferred directly into the uterus where they hopefully implant and begin to develop.

Prospective parents spend countless time and money on trying to have a child. Perhaps the greatest difficulty is the emotional toil it takes and the impact this has on the relationship and on the physical health of the couple. A contributing factor in nearly 50 percent of infertility is problems with the sperm reaching the egg. In men with low sperm motility, many of the sperm cannot swim well enough to reach the egg. A mixture of honey and royal jelly can help with this. Couples experiencing infertility due to low sperm motility were divided into two groups. One group applied a mixture of Egyptian bee honey and royal jelly intravaginally around the time of ovulation and had regular intercourse. The other group underwent intrauterine insemination. After each cycle, 8 percent of couples using the honey and royal jelly mixture became pregnant. Less than 3 percent of couples undergoing intrauterine insemination became pregnant.[104] The results were statistically significant and suggest that using honey and royal jelly in this way may be a better, easier, and more cost-effective way to get pregnant.

59. INFLAMMATION

When the body suffers a physical injury or is under attack from viruses, bacteria, or other pathogens, the immune system reacts to protect and heal the body. What results is inflammation, or swelling of bodily tissue. In acute inflammation (almost immediate swelling), the immune system dispatches white blood cells to the area, which causes the tissue to become hot, red, swollen, and often painful. Mobility may be decreased in the region. This type of inflammation lasts a short while and resolves on its own. Chronic inflammation is longer lasting and can develop over years of trying to battle toxins, pathogens, or even body tissue, as is the case with autoimmune disorders. Tissues affected are often internal, so the symptoms manifest differently from acute inflammation. Some include joint pain, fatigue, fever, digestive troubles, weight gain around the middle, allergies, and skin problems. This type of inflammation can lead to widespread disease in the body like arthritis or cancer. Treatments often use nonsteroidal anti-inflammatory drugs and corticosteroids (cortisone-like medications used to provide relief) to reduce swelling and pain.

Because inflammation and the diseases it causes are often chronic, the use of medications is long-term. Side effects are common. Stomach ulcers, kidney problems, blood pressure changes, worsening of asthma symptoms, and increased risk of stroke and heart attack are some of the more serious ones. A safe and natural alternative is to use honey, which was discovered in a study of rats testing the effectiveness of honey in reducing inflammation in their paws. Rats were given either Malaysian Gelam honey or indomethacin, a nonsteroidal anti-inflammatory drug used to treat pain. Honey was able to significantly reduce the inflamed rat paw and the production of inflammatory chemicals. Results were similar with the indomethacin.[105]

Instead of taking side-effect ridden medication for inflammation, try daily doses of honey. Be sure to monitor your symptoms, and check in with your doctor, especially if inflammation is severe or debilitating.

60. INSOMNIA

A good night's sleep is essential to maintain health and be productive, social, and happy. Most adults require seven to eight hours a night, although the requirement differs from person to person. Having difficulty falling asleep or staying asleep is called insomnia, and this frustrating condition affects many people at various points throughout their lives. Insomnia can be acute and last only a night or a week, or it can be chronic and plague the sufferer for a month or longer.

HEALTH

WELL-BEING

BEAUTY

HOME

Stress, poor sleep habits, jet lag, night shifts, eating too much at night, medications, caffeine, nicotine, alcohol, and medical conditions may be responsible for keeping the mind and body from falling into a deep and restful slumber. Changing personal habits often improves insomnia. Short-term use of sleeping pills may also help, but they tend to lose their effectiveness over time. Yoga, meditation, and acupuncture promote relaxation and can be practiced before bedtime to induce sleepiness.

Honey has been used for centuries to ease the mind and body into a restful nighttime sleep. In Ayurveda, it is mixed with milk, ghee (a type of butter), dates, and spices, but simply adding it to warm water is also beneficial. Honey contains fructose and glucose, which raise insulin levels slightly. This allows tryptophan, an amino acid known to make us sleepy, to enter our brains more easily. In the brain, tryptophan is used in the production of melatonin, a hormone that controls our sleep and wake cycles. It is high at night to induce sleepiness and undetectable in blood levels during the day. Taking a spoonful of honey before bed can coax the body into a sustained and restful sleep.

61. ITCHY SKIN

Itchy skin can be very uncomfortable and make you want to scratch. Itches can be localized to a specific area or generalized and occur all over the body. One of the most common causes is simply having dry skin, and this is easily improved by adding moisture with creams, lotions, and oils. Other causes cannot be resolved so easily. These include itches from allergic reactions, medications, diseases, emotional issues, and skin conditions like eczema.

Sometimes itchy skin is accompanied by bumps, rashes, blisters, or red and inflamed skin. Scratching the itch provides temporary relief but can injure the skin, causing it to look red and raw and, in some cases, become inflamed and bleed. This can lead to infection. Anti-itch creams and lotions can temporarily dull the itch, or cold compresses can briefly quiet the nerve fibers because the sensations of coldness and itchiness travel along the same nerves.

Many treatments do not provide patients with adequate relief from itch and produce significant side effects. When itch results from a rash or irritated skin, honey can be used to suppress the sensation. A study in patients with inflammatory rashes in their skin folds were given either honey or zinc oxide ointment for twenty-one days. Both were effective in treating the rashes, but honey proved to be much better in lowering complaints of itchy skin.[106]

The next time an itchy rash breaks out on the skin, apply a layer of honey. Not only will it lessen the need to scratch the itch, but also it will help heal the rash and reduce the risk of infection.

62. LEAD POISONING

Lead is a heavy metal naturally found in the earth's crust and is widespread in the air, water, and even some homes due to human activities. Manufacturing processes, the burning of fossil fuels, and the use of lead-based products have all increased human exposure to this metal. Lead can be absorbed into the body upon contact and can cause irreparable harm, especially to children. Although symptoms are not usually detected until blood levels are quite high, a blood test can determine the presence of lead in the body so that actions can be taken before it's too late.

In children, lead affects the brain and nervous system and can cause developmental delays, learning difficulties, fatigue, irritability, weight loss, and even seizures. One of the leading ways children are exposed to lead is through eating lead-based paint chips often found in older homes. Other ways include eating and drinking contaminated food and water, eating off of dishware containing lead, or eating soil. Adults are also at risk and may experience headaches, joint pain, muscle pain, memory problems, and high blood pressure. Sperm count in men may be reduced, and pregnant women may miscarry or give birth prematurely.

The first step in combating lead poisoning is to remove the source of lead in the environment. This may include painting over old, lead-based paint or changing dishware to lead-free brands. For more severe cases, chelation therapy is warranted. This is an oral or injectable medication that binds with lead in the body and excretes it in the urine.

Honey has neuroprotective effects against lead and can be consumed to help reduce brain and nervous-system damage in people exposed to this heavy metal. It likely works by increasing antioxidant activities, which protect tissues from oxidative damage that can lead to cognitive decline and chronic inflammation. Male rats exposed to lead had an increase in memory deterioration and anxiety, as well as a decrease in antioxidant activities. When honey was administered with the lead, memory function and antioxidant activities were improved and anxiety decreased.[107] Lead can elevate blood pressure, but honey can lower it. Honey supplemented to hypertensive rats markedly reduced high systolic blood pressure,[108] the most common type of high blood pressure in older people.

63. MENOPAUSAL SYMPTOMS

Menopause is the time in a woman's life when her ovaries no longer produce eggs and menstruation stops. It is a gradual process and is diagnosed when menstrual cycles have ceased for twelve consecutive months. It usually happens when a woman reaches her forties or fifties, although the average age of onset is fifty-one. During this time, a woman experiences many uncomfortable, and sometimes distressing, symptoms. It begins with irregular periods, then hot flashes, night sweats, vaginal dryness, mood changes, insomnia, weight gain, and thinning hair. A few lucky women don't experience any of these symptoms, but most are affected by some, if not all.

Menopause begins when the levels of reproductive hormones begin to decline. This happens naturally with age. A total hysterectomy (which removes the uterus and ovaries) can bring on menopause abruptly. Chemotherapy and radiation therapy for cancer treatment can induce menopause, but this is sometimes reversible. To relieve symptoms, hormone therapy to boost estrogen and progestin levels is effective, but long-term use may increase cardiovascular and breast cancer risks. Medications normally used to treat depression, seizures, and high blood pressure have also proven to provide some relief from some of the symptoms of menopause.

There are natural foods and herbs that have been used to try to alleviate menopausal symptoms. Plant estrogens found in soy, lentils, flaxseed, legumes, and whole grains are often promoted, as are black cohosh and sage. Their effectiveness is largely unproven, but some women find them effective. Honey is another food that is used and has several studies to back it up. Women with breast cancer who are treated with antihormonal drugs often experience menopausal symptoms. When these patients consumed honey, 68 percent reported significant improvement in hot flashes, night sweats, mood changes, insomnia, and vaginal dryness.[109] In another study, postmenopausal women who consumed tualang honey for sixteen weeks improved their immediate memory, a result comparable to women receiving estrogen plus progestin therapy.[110] Tualang honey prevented uterine degeneration, increased bone density, and prevented an increase in body weight when administered to female rats who had their ovaries removed.[111]

The symptoms of menopause are important complications that make daily life difficult for many women, and resolving these or lessening the symptoms can improve self-image and long-term health. Consuming honey is an easy way to find that relief.

64. PINK EYE

Conjunctivitis, or pink eye, is an infection of the clear tissue over the white part of the eye and the lining of the eyelid. When the blood vessels in the whites of the eye become inflamed, they are more visible, and the result is a reddish or pink-looking eye. The eyes may burn, itch, blur, and tear. They often produce a yellow discharge that crusts over the eyelashes and prevents the eye from opening after sleep. The infection can affect one eye or both and is commonly caused by bacteria, viruses, allergens, or irritants. Bacterial and viral pink eye are contagious, so it's important to keep hands away from the eyes to prevent the spread of the infection. Antibiotics are prescribed for bacterial infections, but viral ones have to run their course without the help of medicine. Both types tend to resolve within a week. Pink eye caused by allergens or irritants can clear when the source of infection has been identified and removed.

It may seem unorthodox to put a sweet and sticky substance in the eye, but diluting raw honey with distilled water produces a liquid solution with plenty of antibacterial and anti-inflammatory potency. In fact, a 30 percent solution of honey was found to be effective in inhibiting the growth of bacteria that cause pink eye. Redness, swelling, pus discharge, and duration of infection were all reduced.[112] Another study tested the potency of stingless bee honey in animals with pink eye, and results were similar to those found using the antibiotic gentamicin.[113]

Diluted raw honey drops applied to the eye several times a day may be a good solution to eliminate pink eye in those wanting a safe, natural, and easily accessible remedy.

65. PSORIASIS

Psoriasis is a common skin condition caused when skin cells grow ten times faster than normal. This overabundance of cells creates raised, red plaques with silvery scales on the surface of the skin. These patches can be itchy and painful, and the skin can dry, crack, and bleed. Nails can also become pitted and discolored. Up to 30 percent of people with psoriasis also have psoriatic arthritis and experience pain and swelling in their joints.

Most cases of psoriasis go through periods of flare-up and remission and can be triggered by stress, certain medications, infection, skin injury, smoking, or cold weather. These triggers send a faulty immune system into action. Some of the body's white blood cells attack healthy skin cells, provoking other immune responses that cause the excess of skin cells, redness, inflammation, and other symptoms. There is no cure, but psoriasis can be managed with topical treatments, light therapy, and oral or injectable drugs.

To date, the best that can be hoped for in those with psoriasis is to keep the condition in remission as long as possible and to treat the symptoms of flare-up as they occur. Honey has been shown to be effective in reducing redness, itch, and scaling and thickening of the skin at the site of lesions. In patients treated with a mixture of equal parts honey, olive oil, and beeswax, 62 percent of patients saw significant improvements in their condition. When the honey mixture replaced three quarters of the dose of a topical corticosteroid treatment, 75 percent of patients showed no deterioration in their skin conditions.[114] This means for most individuals, the dose of steroid medications can be reduced (without comprising potency of the treatment) by adding honey to the ointment.

66. REHYDRATION

When the body is in need of water, it is dehydrated. It is important to drink liquids to restore lost water from the body so that normal functions can be carried out. Children and older adults are most at risk of dehydration. One of the leading causes is diarrhea and vomiting. Others include diuretic medications (which cause increased passing of urine) and health conditions that induce the body to lose more water than is taken in. Sweat from vigorous exercise or hot weather can release large quantities of water and metabolites too. Adults may feel dizzy, tired, confused, extremely thirsty, and urinate less often. The urine in dehydrated individuals is often dark yellow. It's a little more difficult to detect dehydration in children. Look out for dry mouth, a lack of tears, the absence of wet diapers for three hours, and a listless or irritable demeanor. It is important to rehydrate as soon as possible to avoid serious complications, including urinary and kidney problems, hypovolemic (low blood volume) shock, and seizures.

Many people opt to rehydrate with plain water or sports drinks. After regular exercise, water is probably adequate. At other times, adding nutrients and electrolytes to the fluid can help the body absorb the liquid more quickly. This is advantageous when dehydration is moderate. Honey contains sugars and small amounts of electrolytes. Adding honey to water provides all the ingredients needed to quickly absorb and replenish much needed fluid and nutrients. Children that were suffering from the stomach flu and given an oral rehydration solution that contained honey reduced their recovery time and showed normal hydration sooner than those children that drank the rehydration solution without the addition of honey.[115] In athletes performing vigorous exercise, rehydration with a honey drink versus plain water improved glucose metabolism and enhanced performance when the athletes were allowed to return to exercise after two hours.[116]

Adding honey to water is recommended as a simple rehydration method that assists the body in recovering more quickly.

HEALTH

WELL-BEING

BEAUTY

HOME

67. ROSACEA

Rosacea is a very common skin condition mostly affecting people of Celtic or Scandinavian descent. It strikes most often in middle age and is characterized by reddened skin that begins in the middle of the face and extends outward. The face, ears, chest, and back may be affected. There are four types of rosacea, some more pronounced than others. Besides skin redness, other symptoms include acne; thick, bumpy skin; and red, irritated eyes. These signs can lead to low self-esteem, anxiety, depression, social withdrawal, and absence from work.

What exactly causes rosacea is not entirely known, but scientists believe this condition runs in families and also can be brought on by environmental triggers that may provoke the immune system into reacting. The presence of the bacteria *H. pylori* or the skin mite called *Demodex* may also play a role. Doctors often prescribe medications to reduce skin redness, acne, inflammation, or bacterial infections. Identifying and eliminating triggers can prevent flare-ups. Protecting the skin from the sun, treating the skin gently, and applying makeup to mask the redness are other options to manage rosacea.

Because of the impact skin conditions can have on a person's quality of life, finding ways to reduce the appearance of redness, acne, and bumps will benefit the individual immensely. Honey has been found to be effective for many with the rosacea condition. Patients diagnosed with rosacea were randomly allocated to receive either a 90 percent medical-grade honey solution or a control cream. After eight weeks, 34 percent of patients in the honey group saw improvements in their skin condition, compared to only 17 percent in the control group.[117]

This simple and easy-to-find solution can be found in most kitchens. Mix the honey with glycerine in a 9:1 ratio and apply to the skin twice a day.

68. SEASONAL ALLERGIES

Allergies can strike in spring when pollen fills the air, at a friend's house when their cute ginger kitten rubs against your leg, or after eating the most satisfying lunch at the local popular seafood restaurant. Allergic reactions can cause minor irritations that result in a stuffy nose, watery eyes, or a mild headache, or they can potentially be so severe as to threaten life. They happen when the immune system reacts to a substance, whether it's swirling through in the air, absorbed through the skin, or eaten for lunch. While these substances don't cause a problem for most people, the immune system of someone with an allergy sees the trigger substance as an unwelcome invader and launches an attack against it. Specific antibodies are produced for each allergen that identify it as harmful to the body. Every time a person comes in contact with that allergen, the allergic response is activated.

There is no cure for allergies, but there are many over-the-counter and prescription drugs available to help ease symptoms. Among these are antihistamines, decongestants, and corticosteroids (cortisone-like medications used to provide relief). They can cause drowsiness, high blood pressure, insomnia, irritability, restricted urine flow, muscle weakness, fluid retention, and weight gain—and these are just some of the side effects. This seems like trading one set of symptoms for another.

For relief from seasonal allergies, some allergy sufferers consume local honey that contains pollen and use it as they would an allergy shot—and they may be on to something. In a study of patients with a physician-diagnosed birch pollen allergy, consuming honey with birch pollen added to it reduced total symptoms by 60 percent compared to patients using only their usual allergy medications. The honey group had twice as many symptom-free days and 70 percent fewer days with severe symptoms. Antihistamine use was reduced by 50 percent.[118] Honey can also extend these effects for up to a month after honey consumption ends.[119]

Consuming honey (especially local if available) on a daily basis, starting before seasonal allergies begin, can provide relief from symptoms and reduce the need for antihistamine medications.

69. SINUS INFECTION

The hollow air spaces within the bones around the nose are the sinuses. When they become swollen and inflamed, sinusitis develops. The tissues produce thick yellow or green mucus, which drains into the nose or down the back of the throat. Breathing through the nose becomes difficult, and there may be pain, pressure, or tenderness around the eyes or nose that worsens when bending over. Sometimes the pain extends to the ears, jaws, and teeth.

Acute sinusitis begins as a cold and usually resolves itself within ten days. Chronic sinusitis lasts for at least twelve weeks and may be caused by allergies, respiratory-tract infections, diseases, or nasal problems. Corticosteroids (cortisone-like medications used to provide relief) or antibiotics are sometimes given to reduce inflammation and destroy the infection (if bacterial).

Bacterial biofilms from *Staphylococcus aureus* are important factors in the development and progression of sinusitis. Biofilms are difficult to destroy because the bacterial cells adhere to each other and mucosal surfaces in a slimy mass. Honey, however, has been found to be effective in killing this pathogen, even in its resistant form. Honey proved to be significantly more effective at removing *Staphylococcus aureus* than commonly used antibiotics.[120] Using honey clears the infection and allows the sinuses to heal.

Oftentimes, sinusitis is chronic due to a deviated septum, infection, or nasal polyps. In some of these cases, functional endoscopic sinus surgery is needed. A thyme-honey nasal spray used after sinus surgery, along with standard medication, reduced inflammation and promoted healing to a greater degree than those patients receiving only the standard medication. Synechiae formation—when two sides in the nasal cavity stick together and obstruct breathing—and nosebleeds were also lower in the thyme-honey treatment group.[121]

To add honey into your at-home treatment for sinusitis, a honey nasal spray can be misted directly into the nostrils or honey can be added to hot water and the steam inhaled.

70. SORE THROAT

A sore throat is pain, irritation, and itchiness of the throat that worsens upon swallowing. The glands of the neck might be swollen or the voice hoarse, and small, white patches can even appear on the tonsils. The main culprits are viral and bacterial infections, but smoke, dry air, and allergies can cause a sore throat as well. When the tissues lining the throat become irritated or infected, blood rushes to the area and brings with it germ-fighting cells. The blood vessels in the tissues swell, putting pressure on the nerve endings and causing pain. Sore throats from viral infections usually last five to seven days and are treated with over-the-counter pain relievers. Bacterial infections, like strep throat, often require antibiotics.

Every infection is different, and the severity and duration of a sore throat depends on the vigor of the particular pathogen, as well as the immune system of the afflicted. One very effective way to soothe a sore throat is to drink honey water. Melt a teaspoon of raw honey in half a cup of warm water (no more than 95 degrees Fahrenheit [35 degrees Celsius]) and slowly sip, allowing the water to wash over the tonsils before swallowing. The honey coats the throat, providing a measure of pain relief from sensitive tissues touching each other during swallowing. Honey also has anti-inflammatory properties and antimicrobial properties to assist the immune system in fighting the infection and returning the swollen tissues to normal. Mixing equal amounts of honey with ginger or lime juice is also said to help. This can be done every few hours, as needed.

71. STREP THROAT

Strep throat is a common bacterial infection of the throat and tonsils. The symptoms come on very suddenly and cause a sore, red, inflamed throat with white patches or tiny red spots on the back of the roof of the mouth. Strep throat is often accompanied by a fever, tender lymph nodes, and headache. *Streptococcus pyogenes*, or group A streptococcus, is the bacteria responsible for this contagious infection. It is spread when a healthy person inhales contaminated air droplets from the cough or sneeze of an infected person. It can also be acquired from sharing food or drinks. Even touching surfaces can pick up the bacteria and cause illness if the bacteria are transferred to the mouth, nose, or eyes. Once transmitted, it takes two to five days for symptoms to develop. **As long as symptoms are present, the infection is contagious.** Oral antibiotics are prescribed to shorten the duration of the illness, reduce the risk of spreading the infection to other parts of the body, and prevent the spread of the bacteria to other people.

The antibacterial activity of honey works very well on group A streptococcus and can be useful in helping the body overcome the infection causing strep throat. Willow herb, heather, and buckwheat honeys from Finland showed significant antimicrobial activity against this group of bacteria.[122] Even when the streptococcus bacteria form difficult-to-eliminate biofilms (slimy masses of bacteria that adhere to each other and other surfaces), honey can benefit. Manuka honey, known for its potent antibacterial activity, was able to cause extensive cell death in group A streptococcus bacteria. It inhibited the ability of the bacteria to adhere to host cells and prevented their invasion.[123]

Consuming honey each day may reduce the risk of developing strep throat by eliminating the bacteria before infection takes hold, or it can be used to assist the body in overcoming the infection by attacking the bacteria directly.

72. TONSILLECTOMY PAIN

The tonsils are a pair of oval-shaped tissues located on either side of the back of the throat. Their function is to help fight infections, and they are a first line of defense when bacteria and viruses enter the mouth. The tonsils are susceptible to infection, especially in children whose immune systems are still developing. The tonsils become red and swollen, and swallowing is painful. These infections often resolve on their own, but some children experience recurrent bouts and need to have their tonsils removed. In other cases, tonsils are naturally enlarged and obstruct breathing, disrupt sleep, and make swallowing a challenge. The person may opt for a tonsillectomy (surgical removal of the tonsils) to eliminate these effects. Surgery itself often takes thirty to forty-five minutes under general anesthesia in an outpatient setting. Recovery takes about ten days, and some of the most common complaints are throat pain and pain that transfers to the ear, jaw, and neck.

After surgery, it is important to rest and drink clear fluids right away. Eating soft foods is encouraged as soon as the patient feels able. To manage pain, doctors prescribe pain medication based on patient age and severity of the pain. Honey can be consumed immediately after tonsillectomy surgery and can help in the recovery period to lessen pain and speed recovery. Patients who had their tonsils removed and were given honey, in addition to acetaminophen (Tylenol) and antibiotics, had significantly less postoperative pain and needed fewer painkillers in the first few days following surgery, compared to a group that only received antibiotics and acetaminophen.[124] The addition of tualang honey for seven days into the diets of post-tonsillectomy patients enhanced the healing of tissue[125] and can be added to the standard regimen of antibiotics in the recovery process. Another study using tualang honey noted that honey consumption reduced the frequency of waking up at night and lowered the use of other pain medications.[126]

Honey, especially tualang honey, is accessible and a low-cost addition to doctor-prescribed treatments that can speed healing and reduce pain after a tonsillectomy.

73. TOOTH DECAY

The mouth is full of bacteria. Some are helpful and others are harmful. The harmful bacteria form a sticky, colorless substance that adheres to the teeth and gum line. This is called plaque. Plaque loves to feed on sugars and starches, so nearly every meal provides plaque with fuel for growth. As the bacteria in the plaque feed on the sugars, they produce acids, which demineralize the tooth surface by extracting calcium and phosphate from the enamel. Saliva tries to neutralize the acids and provide the missing minerals so teeth enamel can remineralize, but sometimes demineralization happens faster than remineralization, and the tooth begins to decay, creating holes or cavities. Cavities are a major oral health concern and affect up to 90 percent of schoolchildren and the majority of adults. The only treatment for cavities is to drill out the decay and fill the hole with composite resins, porcelain, or amalgams.

Once a cavity has begun, the process cannot be reversed. The best course of action is to prevent tooth decay before it starts. A good oral hygiene routine is essential and should involve flossing and brushing twice daily. Reducing sugar consumption can also help to lower acid output from bacteria that cause enamel erosion.

Though a sweet substance, honey doesn't affect the acidity of the mouth like sugar does. Orthodontic patients that chewed honey showed a drop in the acidity of their oral cavity after five minutes, but it did not go low enough to allow demineralization of the enamel. Patients that rinsed their mouths with a sucrose (sugar) solution had acidity levels that did allow demineralization. The period to recover normal acid levels in the mouth was also much quicker with honey than with sugar. The amounts of plaque-forming bacteria in the mouth were also significantly reduced in the honey group.[127]

The exceptionally high antibacterial activity of manuka honey makes it useful as part of a daily oral hygiene regimen. One study found that children who applied manuka honey to their teeth and tongue twice a day, along with regular tooth brushing, had significant reductions in bacteria that contribute to tooth decay when compared to children who did not use honey.[128] Swishing honey around the mouth may protect the teeth by eliminating harmful bacteria in the mouth.

74. VOMITING

Vomiting is the forceful expulsion of the contents of the stomach. It may happen only once or continuously over a short period. The main concern with vomiting is dehydration, particularly in infants and children. A lot of fluid is lost and must be replaced to prevent confusion, headache, and fatigue, or more harmful complications like kidney problems, low blood volume, or seizures.

While indigestion, excessive alcohol consumption, motion sickness, pregnancy, chemotherapy, and some diseases can induce vomiting episodes, most vomiting is caused from bacterial or viral infections in the digestive tract. Occasional throwing up doesn't usually require any treatment, but frequent vomiting or vomiting due to infection is sometimes treated with antiemetic drugs.

It is very distressing when children are sick and vomiting. Being able to prevent vomiting or reduce its frequency would provide immense physical and emotional relief to the family. Solid foods are not recommended, but drinking clear liquids are. Dissolving honey into water or juice can help speed recovery and increase hydration. When children with the stomach flu were given an oral rehydration solution, either with or without the addition of honey, those children who drank the honey solution reduced their vomiting episodes compared to the children not consuming honey in their drink.[129] The honey likely helped eliminate the bacteria or virus responsible for the illness and more quickly rehydrated the body, allowing for a speedier recovery. Consuming honey during recurrent vomiting would benefit adults as well.

75. WARTS

Warts are small skin growths caused by the human papillomavirus (HPV). The warts are usually flesh-colored and contain small black dots, which are actually clotted blood vessels. The hands and the fingers are the most common areas where they are found, which is not surprising since the virus is contagious. If warts occur on the soles of the feet, they are called plantar warts. Most warts go away on their own, but it may take a year or two. Many people find them embarrassing and opt to get rid of them using salicylic acid medications, freezing, or laser treatments. These can cause pain, blistering, and scarring.

Over-the-counter and doctor-administered treatments can be expensive and painful, not to mention ineffective or slow to work. Easy-to-apply home treatments, like honey, can painlessly remove warts. Even children will not object to this method because of its painless application. Apply a thin layer of a medical-grade honey, like manuka, over the wart. Cover it with a bandage or gauze. Repeat this in the morning and evening, leaving the honey in place until the next dressing change. You should see a gradual change in the shape and texture of the wart. Eventually it will disappear. The antimicrobial activity of the honey may be partly responsible for reducing the viability of the virus.

76. WEIGHT LOSS

Having too much body fat increases the risk of health problems like diabetes, heart disease, and certain cancers. Losing weight can improve or prevent any weight-induced conditions. Fat accumulates on the body when more calories are eaten than burned. The body stores these excess calories as fat. Exercising and eating a healthy diet with appropriate calorie intake will help burn the stored fat and reduce body weight. Metabolic processes that occur during times when fat-tissue deposition in the body is increasing can also lead to chronic, low-grade inflammation.

The high consumption of sweeteners contributes to the prevalence of obesity in North America. Honey is different. Although honey is high in fructose and glucose, it evokes a different response in the body than other sweeteners. This was tested in a population of healthy, nonobese women. They were divided into two groups and fed either a meal containing honey or a meal containing sucrose (sugar). The women consuming honey had increases in the hormone peptide YY, which is responsible for reducing appetite. After eating, they also had a delay in activation of the ghrelin response; ghrelin, a hormone, signals hunger to the brain and increases food cravings.[130] The suppression of appetite by honey reduced calorie consumption and protected against weight gain. This idea is supported by a study in two groups of rats fed the same diet with the exception of carbohydrate content. One group had clover honey included in their diet, while the other had an equal amount of sucrose (sugar). After thirty-three days, the rats fed honey had a 14.7 percent lower weight gain. The hormone leptin was also lower by nearly 22 percent; this means that the amount of body fat in the honey-fed rats was lower.[131]

Consuming honey in place of other sweeteners can decrease appetite and reduce calorie intake, body fat, and weight gain.

77. WOUND HEALING

Skin wounds happen to everyone. Whether it's slicing the tip of the finger while dicing carrots or slipping on gravel and scraping a knee, cuts and scrapes tear the skin tissue and often cause bleeding. If the wound is deep, bleeds heavily, or has an object embedded in it, seek medical attention. If it's minor, however, it can be addressed at home. Wash your hands with soap and water. Clean the cut or

HEALTH

WELL-BEING

BEAUTY

HOME

scrape by pouring cool, clean water over it to remove dirt and debris. Then wash with soap and water. Once clean, an antibiotic ointment can be applied.

Sometimes treatments are ineffective, costly, or difficult to access. Honey is none of these. It produces amazing results for wounds: it speeds healing time; it can reduce swelling, pain, odor, and pus; and it can flush out bacteria and prevent infection. It has even been shown to be as effective, or more effective than, standard treatments.

Intrasite Gel is an effective treatment often used to promote wound healing. When compared to honey, healing times of shallow wounds were similar. The average cost of the honey, however, was many times cheaper.[132] In patients with pressure ulcers, honey proved to heal tissue four times more quickly than standard dressing after five weeks of use.[133] In skin-graft patients, honey reduced pain and had similar wound healing times as hydrocolloid dressings.[134] It also reduced odor and improved healing equally as well as silver-coated bandages in patients with malignant wounds.[135] Weekly dressings of manuka honey over leg ulceration wounds for four weeks also reduced wound size, pain, and wound odor.[136]

Honey is an effective, cost-efficient, easy-to-find treatment for the ever-common skin wounds. Simply spread high quality honey over the wound and cover with a bandage or other sterile wrapping.

CHAPTER 3

SALVAGE HAIR AND SKIN

78. ACNE

Acne is a skin condition that results in pimples, blackheads, white-heads, cysts, nodules, and papules. It often appears on the face but can also show up on the neck, chest, back, upper arms, shoulders, and buttocks. Acne is the most common skin problem in the United States. It happens when dead skin cells stick together with sebum (oil) inside the pore and become trapped. Bacteria living on the skin can sometimes get stuck in the pores with the dead skin cells. This provides a perfect breeding ground, and the bacteria quickly multiply. The skin then becomes inflamed.

If the acne goes deeper into the skin, a painful nodule (solid bump) or cyst (pus-filled bump) forms.

Typically, acne appears in teenagers and young adults, but it can affect anyone, even babies. Scars and dark spots on the skin can result. Mild acne can be treated with over-the-counter products that contain benzoyl peroxide or salicylic acid. It takes four to eight weeks of using the product for acne to clear. For best resolution, a dermatologist should treat more severe cases. Prescription-grade topical treatments, whole body treatments like antibiotics, or office procedures involving lasers, lights, or chemicals may be used.

The two types of skin bacteria that cause most acne are *Propionibacterium acnes* and *Staphylococcus epidermidis*. A combination of honey and an extract of cinnamon bark proved to be an effective antibacterial against these two. When used together, honey and cinnamon had an additive effect that greatly reduced bacterial counts.[137] Honey also has anti-inflammatory activity and may help reduce swelling and redness of acne, along with associated pain.

HONEY CINNAMON MASK

1 tablespoon raw honey

1 teaspoon ground cinnamon

1. Mix the two ingredients.
2. Apply a layer of the solution over a clean, dry face. Be sure to avoid the eye area.
3. Leave the honey solution in place for 20 minutes; then wash it off with mild soap.
4. Repeat every day with fresh ingredients. A gradual improvement in skin condition and the disappearance of acne should be evident within a few weeks.

79. AGING

The process of getting older involves many changes in the body. Arteries stiffen, bones lose density, memory declines, skin thins, and wrinkles appear. The rate at which these processes take place varies from person to person. Genetics and illness play a role in when and how we age, but our diet and lifestyle significantly impact the process. There are many theories about aging, but the free-radical theory is growing in popularity as an explanation. It is thought that free radicals are responsible for age-related damage of cells and tissues. Free radicals are unstable molecules actively looking for an electron. They attack the nearest stable molecule and steal one of their electrons, making that molecule a free radical as well. This begins a chain reaction of creating free radicals that ultimately can destroy the cell.

The key to stopping these free radicals lies in the presence of antioxidants. Honey contains antioxidants, one of which is chrysin.

The application of chrysin to adult human skin cells exposed to ultraviolet light (UV) reduces the production of free radicals known as reactive oxygen species. This results in fewer cell deaths. Of note, chrysin is also an anti-inflammatory agent and is able to reduce the expression of inflammatory compounds induced by UVA and UVB light.[138] Tualang honey has shown similar effects. Mouse skin cells treated with this honey before exposure to UVB light prevented cell DNA damage.[139]

Even within the body, antioxidants supplied by honey can work toward creating a more stable environment by reducing excess free radicals and limiting or slowing damage to cells, tissues, and organs.

80. CRACKED HEELS

The skin on the heels of the feet can become dry and crack. The tissue around the rim of the heels may thicken, causing calluses. Cracks can occur in the thick calluses, too, especially if there is too much weight bearing down on the fat pads under the heels in the absence of shoe support. Prolonged standing and improper footwear can increase pressure on the heels, forcing them to expand sideways. If the skin is dry, this increased pressure will cause the skin to crack. Some medical or skin conditions as well can dry the skin, leading to this problem. Most cases of cracked heels are just irritating, but if the condition is severe, it may become painful and unsightly.

It's important to wear proper footwear to support the foot and alleviate excessive pressure on the heels. Shoes with thick soles and closed backs are recommended. To repair the heels, begin by debriding the callused tissue to reduce its thickness; some cracks won't heal if this extra, tough skin is not removed. Next, soak the feet in a warm footbath. Immediately after, apply a honey solution to the heels. Honey enables the foot to retain the moisture from the footbath and helps seal it in. This allows the tissue to begin healing. The honey is also antibacterial and can provide protection from pathogens trying to invade through the broken skin.

HONEY REPAIR FOR CRACKED HEELS

1 tablespoon raw honey
1/2 teaspoon milk
1 teaspoon lemon juice

1.   Mix the ingredients together, and apply the paste to the heels.
2.   Leave it on for 30 minutes.
3.   Rinse and pat dry. Repeat daily.

81. DANDRuFF

Dandruff is a chronic condition marked by the flaking of skin cells on the scalp. They are visible as white, oily-looking flakes of skin in the hair and on the shoulders. It is not a dangerous condition, but it can be embarrassing for some people. Dandruff is usually worse in the fall and winter when the scalp is subjected to the drier, cooler outdoor air and heated indoor air, which depletes moisture in the skin. It can be caused by not shampooing enough so that dead skin cells mix with oils. This causes a buildup and subsequent shedding of these cells as dandruff.

Yeast on the scalp can irritate the skin of some people and cause an overproduction of skin cells, which flake off as dandruff. Dry skin can cause smaller, drier flakes to appear. One of the most common causes of dandruff, however, is seborrheic dermatitis. This is a condition in which oily skin is covered in flaky white or yellow scales. Mild cases are easy to treat with daily cleansing to reduce oil and skin-cell buildup. Others cases are more difficult and may need medicated shampoos. Some shampoos contain antifungal and antibacterial agents to kill the microbes. Others work by slowing the death rate of skin cells to reduce buildup and flaking.

Applying a honey-water solution directly to the scalp can help lock in moisture and reduce dry skin that becomes dandruff. It also helps scale down seborrheic dermatitis and improves the condition of the scalp so that skin flaking and dandruff are reduced. When patients with dandruff from seborrheic dermatitis applied honey water to their scalps, itching and scaling (leading to dandruff) were greatly reduced within just one week, and skin lesions were healed after two weeks. The honey treatment continued for six months, with weekly applications. During this time, no relapses were observed in any of the patients.[140]

This simple treatment of honey-water appears to be very effective in reducing dandruff. It can be applied in the privacy of the home with little cost and big convenience.

82. DRY LIPS

Chapped lips are characterized by dry, cracked lips that can be red and itchy. The skin on the lips is very thin and provides only a small measure of protection to the tissue underneath. It does not contain any sebaceous glands to produce moisturizing oil, and water loss from the lips is much higher than anywhere else on the body. Other exacerbating factors include dry environmental conditions, lip licking, sun damage, vitamin deficiencies, medication, and infections. It's easy to see why chapped lips are such a common problem for many.

The first step to achieving smooth, soft lips is to exfoliate with a gentle lip scrub. You can make your own at home with honey, white sugar, jojoba oil, and peppermint essential oil. You can keep the mixture in the bathroom and use it daily or when lips are chapped. It's also important to moisturize the lips and keep them hydrated throughout the day. Honey locks in moisture and provides a protective barrier that allows dry and cracked skin on the lips to heal. You can make lip balm at home with honey, coconut oil, and olive oil mixed together.

If the lip scrub and lip balm are used often, dry lips will heal rapidly, and lip strength and elasticity will increase.

HONEY LIP SCRUB

1 teaspoon honey
2 teaspoons white sugar
1/2 teaspoon jojoba oil
1 drop peppermint essential oil

1. Mix the ingredients in a small glass jar, and keep it in the bathroom for up to one month.
2. Use daily or when lips are chapped.

HONEY LIP BALM

1 teaspoon honey
1 teaspoon coconut oil
1 teaspoon olive oil

1. Put all ingredients together and mix thoroughly. Mixing may be easier to achieve by gently warming the ingredients on the stove.

2. Store in a small glass jar. Apply the lip balm each evening, and leave on for as long as desired.

83. FACIAL CLEANSER

Keeping the skin radiant, moisturized, and blemish-free requires regular cleansing. Facial cleansers come as gels, creams, lotions, foams, powders, clays, or bars. Each is touted to either decongest clogged pores, draw out toxins, remove oil, kill bacteria, moisturize, exfoliate, reduce the signs of aging, or remove makeup. What they all have in common is the ability to remove dirt and oil from the skin, although to varying extents. Most facial cleansers on the market contain a long list of unrecognizable ingredients. While some are beneficial to the skin, many are not. These include synthetic fragrances, detergents, preservatives, and alcohols. These can irritate the skin, clog pores, dry the skin, or even interfere with the normal functioning of the body.

To avoid these issues, many turn to natural products in their skin-care routine. Honey is commonly used to cleanse the skin by removing dirt, oil, and impurities and seal in moisture. It has antibacterial compounds that effectively fight acne-causing bacteria[141] and even works on reducing the symptoms of rosacea.[142] Honey contains antioxidants that protect against UV damage[143] and anti-inflammatory agents to reduce swelling from acne or other skin conditions.

Before using the honey cleanser, remove all makeup. Make sure the face is wet with water and apply about ½ teaspoon of raw honey to the face. Smooth it all over using a circular motion. Additional water may be needed, depending on the consistency of the honey. Leave it in place for about ten minutes, then rinse it off with warm water. Pat dry with a clean towel. Your face should feel clean, plump, moisturized, and soft.

84. HAIR CONDITIONER

There are about one hundred thousand to one hundred fifty thousand hairs on the human head. Those are a lot of strands to take care of. Each strand of hair consists of three layers with the outer layer, or cuticle, protecting the inner two layers. When the hair is healthy, the scales of the cuticle overlap tightly and protect the inner layers. When it becomes damaged, however, the scales of the cuticle loosen and separate, exposing the layers underneath. The hair looks dry and dull and may break easily. The inner layers can become damaged from exposure to the UV rays of the sun, heat, pollution, chlorine, or any of the array of chemicals found in hair products and treatments.

Conditioning the hair seals the cuticle by smoothing down the scales to give a soft, smooth, and healthy appearance to the hair. Conditioning also reduces the stress of towel drying and brushing and helps with detangling. When conditioning, begin a few inches from the scalp and apply toward the ends. The older the hair, the more damaged it likely is. Most conditioners are intended to be used after every shampoo, but others are deep conditioners and work best when used only once or twice a week.

Honey attracts and seals moisture into the cuticle. It also protects against sun-induced damage and provides a barrier to environmental toxins. Honey can be mixed with apple cider vinegar in a 1:2 ratio or with coconut or olive oil in a 1:1 ratio. Mix thoroughly, gently warming the solution if needed. Apply enough to the hair to lightly coat the strands and leave it in for five minutes. This can be done in the shower after shampooing. Rinse it out with warm water. Honey conditioner can be used several times a week for smooth, shiny hair.

85. MOISTURIZER

Having hydrated and moisturized skin gives a healthy glow and a more youthful appearance. Dehydration causes skin cells to build up on the surface, rather than slough off, resulting in a dry, rough appearance. Elasticity is lost, and the skin becomes tight and possibly cracked. Fine lines and wrinkles are more pronounced. Moisture loss can be a result of sun damage, hot showers, wind, excessive consumption of diuretic drinks (like coffee, alcohol, or tea), avoidance of moisturizers, or harsh skin products. It worsens with age due to the decline in oil-gland activity and the lowered ability of the skin to hold onto water.

Rehydrating the top layers of skin and locking in moisture will help improve the appearance and feel of dry skin. Honey draws water into the skin and retains the moisture, providing a plump, youthful appearance in place of dry, flaking, or wrinkled skin. It can be used on all types of skin, even sensitive. Raw honey contains alpha hydroxy acids, which allow dead skin cells to loosen and wash away. This allows new skin cells to rise to the surface and better absorb moisture. These acids also stimulate collagen production and reduce the appearance of fine lines and wrinkles. **Before applying a moisturizer, always wash the face first to prevent sealing in dirt and debris. Failure to do so may result in clogged pores.**

RINSE-OFF HONEY MOISTURIZER

1 teaspoon honey
1/4 teaspoon jojoba oil
1/8 teaspoon lime juice

1. Mix the three ingredients together.
2. Apply over clean, dry skin.
3. Allow it to remain for about 10 minutes, and then gently wipe away with a warm, damp cloth. The honey moisturizer can be used all over the body for soft, smooth skin.

86. NAILS

Nails can become either brittle and dry due to moisture loss, or soft and brittle due to too much moisture. Sometimes disease or diet is the culprit, but more often, external factors are responsible. This is particularly true if the toenails are strong but the fingernails are weak. The constant wetting and drying of the nails through numerous hand washing, dish washing, showers, and chores, not to mention the use of detergents, harsh cleaners, and nail polish removers, all wreak havoc on nail health and can cause irreversible damage. Often, the damaged nails have to be grown out. As the new nails grow in, take care to make sure they remain healthy. Wear gloves when doing chores, moisturize the cuticles, soak the nails in oil, and clip or file them regularly.

Honey makes a great moisturizer and can be used to soften the skin of the cuticles so they can be pushed down and the dead skin clipped away. Honey also works well in removing hangnails. The moisture that honey seals into the skin makes it pliable and the hangnails easy to remove without damaging surrounding skin. Moisturizing the nails once a day with honey can help lock in moisture and sebum produced by the body. Nails can absorb water from the external environment, but it tends to be quickly lost. Oils remain longer and work better than water, so try blending honey with an oil. The honey provides a natural barrier to moisture loss, keeping the added oil and the natural sebum in place longer.

HONEY NAIL LOTION

1 teaspoon honey
1 teaspoon jojoba oil or coconut oil

1. Blend these two ingredients together, and spread the lotion generously over the nail bed and cuticle.
2. Allow this to soak in for about 15 minutes.
3. Wash off with warm water, and apply a leave-on moisturizer.

87. SHAVING CREAM

Shaving creams don't just come as creams; they can be purchased as gels or foams as well. They are often used by men to shave their beards and by women to remove hair from their legs, armpits, and other areas. Shaving with just water and a razor can damage the skin. Nicks and cuts or an itchy, swollen, red rash (known as razor burn) might develop. To prevent this, shaving cream (or gel or foam) is used to hydrate the skin and the hairs. Supple skin is more flexible and can move with the razor. Softer hairs take less force to cut and thereby reduce the risk of nicking the skin. The layer of protection cream provides also reduces friction so that the razor glides over the skin effortlessly. Some of the ingredients are also designed to soothe and refresh the skin.

Many shaving creams contain synthetic colors and fragrances, propylene glycol to keep the skin moist, triethanolamine to keep oils and water emulsified, sodium lauryl sulfate to create lather, and mineral oil to lock in moisture. These can irritate the skin and lungs and clog the pores. In place of commercially available shaving products, try using honey. It can be used on its own or mixed with a small amount of water to reduce viscosity. Simply spread it over the skin and shave it off. It can also be combined with other ingredients and used on any body part. Honey draws water to the skin and locks it in, making the skin resilient and the hair supple. Shaving becomes a smooth and comfortable process that leaves the skin feeling soft.

HONEY SHAVING CREAM

1 tablespoon honey
1 teaspoon almond oil
1 teaspoon aloe vera gel

1. Mix the three ingredients together, and spread over the skin.
2. Using a razor, remove the solution along with the hair.

HEALTH

WELL-BEING

BEAUTY

HOME

88. SPLIT ENDS

The outer layer of the hair shaft is called the cuticle. It is very strong and made up of overlapping layers of protein called keratin. It protects the inner layers and is what gives hair its flexibility and volume. The cuticle can become damaged from chemicals, UV rays, chlorine, heat, or physical stress, such as frequent, vigorous brushing or use of hair extensions. When the cuticle becomes damaged, it can no longer hold the hair shaft together and it splits. Split ends give the appearance of a dry, brittle, frizzy, or untamed mane.

The only way to truly get rid of split ends is to cut away the damaged hair. Moving forward, the key is to prevent split ends before they happen. Honey can be mixed with coconut oil to create a moisturizing hair mask. It attracts and retains water in the hair shaft and seals the cuticle, ensuring long-lasting moisture and protection from dryness that leads to damage.

SPLIT-ENDS REPAIR

2 tablespoons honey
2 tablespoons coconut oil

1. Mix the two together in a bowl.
2. Massage the solution into the last three inches of hair. If you have layers, you may need more to cover all the ends.
3. Loosely tie the hair on top of the head, and wrap the hair in a warm towel for 15 minutes.
4. Rinse off in warm water. The hair should appear smooth, shiny, and hydrated.

· ·

89. SUNBURN

Sitting outside in the sun for too long without the protection from sunscreen can cause the skin to burn. The ultraviolet rays of the sun penetrate the skin and increase the rate of melanin production, the body's way of protecting the skin from the damaging effects of the sun. But when exposure is too long or the rays too intense, melanin is not enough, and it burns. The skin becomes red, painful, and swollen. It is hot to the touch and may form small, fluid-filled blisters.

Tanning lamps can burn the skin in the same way the sun does. Even the sun's rays that reflect off the surface of water, sand, ice, and snow can give a sunburn. Surprisingly, cloudy days still emit 80 percent of the sun's ultraviolet rays, so caution is needed for outdoor activities on these days as well. Sunburned skin begins to heal itself within a few days. Pain relievers and corticosteroids (cortisone-like medications used to provide relief) are often used for pain and to control itching.

While nothing but time can remove a sunburn, the symptoms can be managed with honey. It has been used as a topical burn salve for centuries. Honey speeds up the healing process by stimulating tissue growth and the development of new blood vessels. It reduces pain, itching, redness, and swelling of the damaged skin. A thick layer of honey smoothed over the sunburned area can prevent painful sun blisters from breaking and exposing the damaged and tender tissue underneath. It works by helping to draw the fluid out of the blister. What is left are thickened areas of skin that protect the damaged skin tissue below and seal out bacteria, preventing

HEALTH

WELL-BEING

BEAUTY

HOME

HEALTH

infection. If some of the skin begins to peel or crack, bacteria and other pathogens can enter these areas too. Honey has antimicrobial compounds that are very effective at destroying these.

To achieve the best results when treating your sunburn with honey, make sure to use a high-quality honey that is high in antimicrobial compounds. The processed and ultra-filtered honey found in grocery stores will not work as well.

WELL-BEING

BEAUTY

HOME

CHAPTER 4

INDOORS AND OUTDOORS

90. ALMOND MILK

Milk is a nutritious drink that is enjoyed by many toddlers and children. Some adults are able to drink milk, too, but a majority have difficultly digesting lactose, the main sugar in milk. When they do drink milk, they end up with cramps, gas, bloating, nausea, and sometimes diarrhea. Because of this, alternative plant-based milk drinks have become quite popular, with almond milk at the top of the list.

Almond milk has a creamy texture and a mild, nutty flavor. It contains vitamins and minerals, but it is not as nutritious as cow's milk and is not a suitable substitute for infants. Make sure to purchase unsweetened varieties to avoid unwanted added sugars and calories. Commercially purchased almond milk contains small amounts of gums that are generally safe in limited amounts, but because they are mostly indigestible, they may cause digestive problems for some.

Making almond milk at home can provide a healthy, delicious, additive-free beverage that can be enjoyed by all, even those with sensitive colons. Adding a bit of sweetness with honey not only kicks up the flavor but also adds a boost of antioxidants and nutrients.

ALMOND MILK WITH HONEY

2 cups raw almonds
4 cups water
2 tablespoons raw honey
1 teaspoon vanilla extract

1. Soak the almonds in filtered water overnight. The bowl can be left out on the counter, covered with a cloth. This process allows the almonds to sprout, making them easier to digest. The almonds can be soaked longer for a creamier milk.

2. Remove the almonds from the water, rinse, and place them in a blender.

3. Add 2 cups of water to the almonds, and blend at high speed for 2 to 4 minutes until a smooth paste forms.

4. Add the honey and vanilla, and blend until incorporated.

5. Add the remaining water, and blend for 2 to 3 minutes until the mixture takes on a milky look and texture.

6. Strain the mixture through several layers of cheesecloth to remove the almond solids. These can be used for another purpose.

7. The almond milk is now ready to drink. It only lasts a few days in the refrigerator, so only make what you will use in that period. If a thicker milk is desired, use less water. If thinner is what you're after, use more water.

91. ANTS

There are trillions of ants around the world, so it is no surprise to find them in your garden or home. These social insects live in large numbers, so if you see a few milling around some plants in the backyard or walking across the floor on the way to the pantry, beware. If allowed to go on their merry way, they will arrive in droves and make themselves at home.

There is no beneficial reason for ants to enter your home, but in the garden they are helpful in aerating the soil for plants and controlling some other insect populations. They also serve as food for lizards, birds, spiders, and other insects; however, that's pretty much where their usefulness ends. Ants can wreak havoc in the garden and will eat almost any fruit, vegetable, or plant. To make matters worse, they protect insects that produce honeydew (a sweet, sticky substance) and feed on plants, allowing these insects to thrive and potentially decimate your favorite greenery.

Ant baits and traps can be purchased at grocery and home improvement stores. Many contain insecticides that are linked to a number of health concerns. Since manufacturers are not required to list the inactive ingredients in their ant formulas, the consumer never really knows what they are bringing into their home and exposing their family to. A safe and very effective ant bait that can be made at home to trap and remove ants involves only four ingredients: honey, water, borax, and cotton balls. The honey will attract the ants, and borax will poison them. Borax is a mineral that is toxic to ants and is a mild skin irritant to humans. Gloves should be worn when handling it.

HONEY ANT BAIT

1/4 cup honey
1/2 cup water
2 tablespoons borax
cotton balls

1. Heat the water on the stove over medium-high heat.
2. Stir in the borax and honey until they have both dissolved. Allow the solution to cool.
3. Soak the cotton balls in the liquid.
4. Wearing rubber or latex gloves, remove the cotton balls, and gently squeeze out most of the excess liquid.

5.   Place the cotton balls on a small dish or plastic lid, and place the unit around the house where the ants have been observed.

Ants are drawn to the sweet scent of the cotton ball dipped in the honey and borax solution. The ants will eat the cotton and, along with it, the borax. After 24 to 48 hours, all the ants should be gone.

92. CANNING FRUITS

The process of canning foods began a few hundred years ago as a way to preserve foods for long periods of time without spoiling. The first canning took place in glass jars, sealed with wax, wrapped in canvas, and then boiled. Unbreakable tin cans were subsequently used in place of glass in many places, including the United States, which began to produce unsweetened condensed milk. It was determined that heat was the element needed to preserve food, but it wasn't initially known why. Now we know that bacteria, molds, and yeasts present in air, water, and soil can spoil food. By heating the foods, these organisms are destroyed. This heating process also stops the action of enzymes that break down food and reduce its quality.

One of the most common groups of foods preserved at home is fruits. Because these have high acid content, fruits can easily be preserved in a boiling-water canner. Boiling-water canners can be purchased online, but large metal pots can also be used if they are tall enough to cover the cans or bottles with at least an inch of water. It is best to use jars designed for home canning, as other jars may not be sturdy enough and could break during the process. Just

HEALTH

WELL-BEING

BEAUTY

HOME

about any fruit can be preserved. Choose freshly picked, firm fruits for best results.

HONEY SYRUP PRESERVED PEACHES

1/2 cup honey
8 cups filtered water
12 ripe peaches
8 pint jars

1. Add the peaches to boiling water for 1 minute. Remove and peel the peaches. If the skin doesn't come off easily, add the peaches back to the boiling water for another minute. Alternatively, blanch them in ice-cold water for easier peeling.

2. Slice the peaches into four pieces, and discard the pit.

3. Submerge the jars upside down in the boiling water canner to sterilize them. Leave them in the water until they are ready to use so that they remain hot. Make sure to sterilize the lids and rings as well.

4. Bring the 8 cups of filtered water to a boil, and add the honey. Stir until the honey has melted. Keep the liquid simmering.

5. Remove the jars from the canner and add the peaches to each jar, filling to about an inch below the lid.

6. Pour the honey syrup over the peaches until they are just covered.

7. Remove any air bubbles.

8. Place the lid on the jar, and seal it with the ring.

9. Put the jars into the boiling water canner, making sure the boiling water is at least 1 inch above the jar.

10. After 25 minutes, remove the jars and set aside to cool.

93. FRUIT BROWNING

Preparing cut apples for school lunches or arranging a fruit tray for a party often needs to be done hours in advance. By the time the fruit is eaten, it has turned an ugly shade of brown. While the fruit is perfectly safe to eat, its appearance makes less enticing, and you'll be left with a plateful of leftovers that no one will want. When fruits are peeled or sliced, the cells along the cut lines are torn open. This releases an enzyme from the cells called polyphenol oxidase. When this enzyme is exposed to oxygen in the air, a reaction occurs in which the polyphenol oxidase converts plant phenols into melanin, a dark pigment that turns the flesh of the fruit brown.

To prevent this reaction from happening every time you slice a pear or banana, soak them in honey water for thirty seconds after cutting them. Honey contains a peptide compound that prevents the enzymatic reaction between polyphenol oxidase and oxygen. Browning doesn't occur, and you are left with a beautiful piece of fruit that will keep bright and fresh-looking for hours.

HONEY FRUIT SOAK

1 cup water

2 tablespoons honey

1. Gently heat the water and honey mixture so that the honey completely dissolves.
2. Allow the water to cool to room temperature.
3. Dip cut fruit into the honey water for 30 seconds, and then remove.

94. HONEY TAFFY

Taffy is a sticky, soft candy most often made from sugar or molasses and butter. Other ingredients, including natural and artificial food coloring and flavors, are added to create a wide assortment of delectable treats in every color of the rainbow and every flavor imaginable. From root beer to peppermint, key lime to chocolate hazelnut, the varieties are endless. Most people call the candy "salt water taffy."

This term came into being when an unfortunate event happened to David Bradley, a candy merchant with a stand on Atlantic City's boardwalk in the 1880s. One evening, the ocean waters rose and flooded his candy stand. His supply of taffy was soaked. The next day, a little girl came by and asked for some taffy. He jokingly asked her if she wanted salt water taffy, making fun of the fact that his candy was drenched in Atlantic Ocean salt water. She tried it and loved it. Bradley's mother overheard her son refer to the candy as "salt water taffy" and suggested he keep the name. It stuck.

Salt water taffy is cooked in large copper or stainless steel kettles, cooled, and then pulled repeatedly to add air bubbles. This aeration process keeps the taffy soft. After pulling, the taffy is cut into small pieces and wrapped in wax paper with twists at both ends. They are sold individually and by the pound in specialty confection shops and national chain stores.

Taffy can be made at home, and doing so is a fun experience that can be shared with the whole family. It's really simple and doesn't use any artificial ingredients, fats, or salt. In fact, it only has one ingredient—honey.

SALT WATER TAFFY

1 cup honey

1. Begin by boiling the honey over medium-high heat until it reaches 285 degrees Fahrenheit (141 degrees Celsius). This is when the honey arrives at the soft-crack stage and the sugar concentration of the honey is 95 percent.

2. Pour the honey onto a baking sheet lined with parchment paper that is lightly coated with cooking spray. Spread it out with a spatula and allow it to cool for about 10 minutes.

3. Coat your hands with butter or cooking spray and work the honey into a ball. Pick it up and stretch it into a long strand. Fold the strand back over itself and press the ends together. Repeat this process of pulling and folding until the honey turns a light caramel color.

4. Loosely roll the taffy into a long, thin line (about half an inch thick), and cut into one-inch pieces.

5. Individually wrap each piece in waxed paper, twisting the ends. You now have salt water taffy.

95. LAND SNAILS AND SLUGS

Snails and slugs are bothersome pests in gardens that feed on living plants and decaying matter. They can cause serious damage to seedlings, herbs, and ripening fruit. Each has both eggs and sperm, so they can become quite prolific when conditions are favorable. Snails and slugs can lay hundreds of eggs a year in the soil, beneath

HEALTH

WELL-BEING

BEAUTY

HOME

leaves, and in other protected areas of the garden. They tend to be most active at night and on cloudy days. Other than plant damage, their presence can be identified by a silvery slime trail from the mucus secreted by the body that helps them glide along.

To get rid of snails and slugs, several methods are needed. Eliminate areas where they can hide during the day. Make the habitat less inviting by reducing moisture—use drip irrigation over sprinklers—and invest in snail-proof plants. Copper barriers can be installed around susceptible plants. The copper reacts with the slime and disrupts their nervous system. Then handpick the snails and slugs you see in the garden. At night, put out a snail and slug trap to catch them when they come out of hiding. It's important to place them close to where you believe the slugs are living and feeding because they will not travel too far.

A honey and yeast water trap will attract snails and slugs. They fall into the container and drown, leaving your garden slug- and snail-free.

HONEY YEAST DETERRENT

1/4 cup honey
1/4 cup yeast
4 cups water

1. Gently heat the water over the stove, and add the honey. Stir until it has dissolved. Allow it to cool to lukewarm.
2. Pour the honey water into jam jars, yogurt cups, or any container that is deep enough for the slug to drown.
3. Sprinkle the yeast on top of the water.
4. Place the containers in the soil of the garden so that the top is at ground level. Replace the solution every other day, and discard what is caught.

96. MOIST BAKED GOODS

Cakes, cookies, breads, and pastries can be sweet or savory and enjoyed at any meal, any time of the day. Old and young alike are tempted by these sumptuous foods, and I think we can all agree that they are best when moist and flavorful. I can't think of a single person who prefers a dry, crumbly cake to a soft, spongy one. There are several methods that can add moisture into baked goods or ensure from the beginning they turn out moist. If your cake is too dry, try drizzling a simple honey syrup over it.

SIMPLE HONEY SYRUP

1/2 cup raw honey

1 cup water

1. Heat the water, and melt the honey into it. Allow the solution to cool.
2. Cut the cake in half horizontally, and sprinkle the honey syrup over the cake.
3. Reassemble and allow the cake to sit for several hours. The moisture from the syrup will distribute throughout the cake.

When following a recipe, honey can be substituted for sugar. This adds extra moisture without compromising sweetness. Because honey is sweeter than sugar, however, use ¾ cup of honey in place of 1 cup of sugar to ensure similar sweetness. If desired, honey can be substituted in a 1:1 ratio with sugar. When doing this, reduce another liquid in the recipe by ¼ cup for every cup of honey used. An extra ½ teaspoon of baking soda is also needed to reduce the acidity of the honey and help the food rise as before. The beauty of using honey is that you get to choose your favorite varietal, which lends a unique flavor to the food.

....

97. PET HOT SPOTS

Hot spots, or acute moist dermatitises as your vet will call them, are painful sores that arise when dogs repeatedly lick, chew, scratch, or bite an area of their skin. The skin becomes traumatized and damaged, producing a red, hot, and often oozing lesion. The lesion is itchy and uncomfortable for your dog, and he will continue to bite and scratch it, making it worse.

Some hot spots begin with irritation caused by a bee sting or tick bite, but more often an underlying condition is responsible, such as a flea or food allergy, parasite, skin infection, contact irritant, or skin disease. A veterinarian can be helpful in determining the trigger for hot spots. Most hot spots are not that serious and can be treated at home. If left alone, they can become easily infected with bacteria. This can greatly exacerbate the lesion and cause it to spread.

The first step is to recognize the hot spot. It is commonly found on the head, hips, and chest. Pay attention if you see your dog chewing or licking one particular area of her skin. Sometimes the lesion is hidden under fur and can go undetected for a time. As the hot spot grows worse, the fur around the lesion will wear off. Trim away any fur remaining over and around the wound. If the hot spot is large, the area may need to be shaved. Clean the lesion with mild soap and water. Pat the area dry. Apply a layer of high quality raw honey over the hot spot. If the dog tries to lick the honey off, an Elizabethan collar (also known as a cone) may be needed around his neck.

The honey will reduce redness, inflammation, itching, and pain. It will allow the tissue to begin regeneration and keep the area clean and moist, but protected from bacteria. Reapply the honey as needed until the hot spot has healed.

98. PREBIOTIC

Prebiotics are natural food components that cannot be digested. They are found in a number of foods, including raw honey. Fructo-oligosaccharide is one prebiotic supplied by honey that ferments in the colon and has a number of physiological effects. It increases the number of good bacteria, which improves gastrointestinal health and raises the number of vitamins and digestive enzymes produced. Good bacteria boost the immune system and inhibit the growth of yeasts, bacteria, and other pathogens that can harm health. Fructooligosaccharide is also thought to increase the absorption of calcium to aid in keeping bones and teeth strong. It shortens the duration of time fecal matter takes to move through the colon and also increases the amount of feces produced. This means unwanted or unneeded food components get shunted into the feces, rather than absorbed by the body. Prebiotics may also play a role in lowering blood fat levels.

Honey is known to reduce total cholesterol and triglyceride levels. Perhaps the prebiotics in honey are partly responsible for this.

99. RACCOoNS

Raccoons are wild animals that prefer to live in forested areas with lots of trees, water, and vegetation. Many of them, however, are found in towns and cities where they make their homes in attics, barns, sheds, and even sewers. Highly intelligent and with great dexterity, these animals are able to successfully forage for food right in your backyard. They will eat almost anything they can find, but most of their diet consists of insects and sweet food like fruit. Frogs, snakes, fish, birds' eggs, and nuts are other favorites. If pickings are slim, raccoons will eat whatever is in your trash can. They can pry the lid off trash bins and even open jars and bottles. They are also adept at opening doors, so if you suspect raccoons in the area, make sure your doors are tightly closed and locked at night. The destruction doesn't stop at tipping your trash can. Raccoons can destroy gardens and eat crops, raid bird feeders, and upset beehives. They also carry *Salmonella*, rabies, and roundworm, which can be transferred to pets and humans.

It is safe to say that raccoons are nuisances. If one or a family of raccoons has invaded your space and is wreaking havoc on your property, the best thing to do is to trap them and relocate them (with permission) to private property, in the same county, that has shelter, food, and water available to them. Purchase a large, sturdy steel cage. Set it up on a stable surface, and put a weight on top so that the raccoon doesn't tip it over. Make sure it is not near anything that the raccoon can grab hold of and destroy once he is trapped. He will tend to do this. Bait the trap with marshmallows dipped in honey. The marshmallows can be placed leading up to the trap, with some at the back of the trap. The sweet scent will attract the raccoons, and they will follow the trail of honeyed marshmallows, eating them up as they go. Once caught in the trap, use gloves to move the trap to your vehicle and relocate the raccoon. Licensed wild animal control operators can be called to do this if you don't want to trap the raccoon yourself.

100. SPORTS DRINK

If working out for an hour or less, the best way to hydrate is with water. Prolonged exercise, particularly with a lot of sweating, requires electrolytes, carbohydrates, and fluid to properly replenish the body. Failure to replenish those components may lead to headaches and muscle cramps. There are many commercial sports drinks available to choose from. They all contain water and a long list of vitamins and minerals. This seems good. They can balance out fluids in the body and allow the muscles to function properly. But as you keep reading the ingredients, you'll see preservatives, artificial flavors and colors, and large amounts of sugar. The sugar is intended to not only sweeten the drink, making it desirable for kids and adults alike, but to give the body much needed energy. This energy is quickly depleted, though, and can leave the athlete feeling even more fatigued. In addition, the amount of sugar added is much too high, which can lead to weight gain. After spending all that time exercising to achieve a healthy body, you defeat the purpose with these drinks.

It's easy to make hydrating sports drinks at home that have all of the goodness the body needs and none of the harmful ingredients.

HONEY SPORTS REFRESHER

4 cups filtered water
2 tablespoons raw honey
1/4 teaspoon sea salt
1/4 teaspoon calcium and magnesium powder
1/4 cup orange juice
1/4 cup lemon juice

1. On the stove, gently heat one cup of the water.
2. Add the honey, sea salt, and calcium and magnesium powder. Whisk until everything has dissolved into the water.
3. Remove from the heat, and mix in the remaining ingredients.
4. Pour into a glass container, and keep in the refrigerator.

101. WILTED PLANTS

Potted plants in the house and in-ground plants outside are both susceptible to wilting. This occurs when the plant is not getting enough water. Limited or no water means the plant cannot carry out cellular processes, transport nutrients, or store excess water in its cells. It is actually the storage of water in the vacuoles of the cells that plumps them up. The water pushes against the cell walls, making them rigid and forcing the plant to stand tall and strong. When the plant has to use the water in its vacuoles, the cells shrink, and the pressure against the cell walls decreases. The leaves, stems, and flowers droop and start to turn brown.

To revive wilted plants, use a honey and water solution. It slows the rate of water evaporation from the pores of the leaves. The honey in the water provides a source of nutrients for beneficial bacteria and fungi in the soil, which promotes a healthy root system and enhances plant growth.

PLANT-REVIVING SOLUTION

1 gallon (3.8 liters) water
3 tablespoons honey

1. Mix the water and honey together. The water may need to be warmed a bit to dissolve the honey.
2. When cooled to room temperature, saturate the soil of the plant (in the sink, if potted, to allow for drainage).
3. Spray a mist of the water onto the leaves every other day.

HEALTH

WELL-BEING

BEAUTY

HOME

NOTES

1. A. Hocaoglu Babayigit, "High Usage of Complementary and Alternative Medicine among Turkish Asthmatic Children," *Iranian Journal of Allergy, Asthma and Immunology* 14, no. 4 (August 2015): 410–15.
2. Nurfatin A. Kamaruzaman, Siti A. Sulaiman, Gurjeet Kaur, and Badrul Yahaya, "Inhalation of Honey Reduces Airway Inflammation and Histopathological Changes in a Rabbit Model of Ovalbumin-Induced Chronic Asthma," *BMC Complementary and Alternative Medicine*, 14 (2014): 176, https://bmccomple mentalternmed.biomedcentral.com/articles/10.1186/1472-6882-14-176.
3. A. N. Fauzi, Mohd N. Norazmi, and Nik S. Yaacob, "Tualang Honey Induces Apoptosis and Disrupts the Mitochondrial Membrane Potential of Human Breast and Cervical Cancer Cell Lines," *Food and Chemical Toxicology* 49, no. 4 (2011): 871–78.
4. Nik S. Yaacob, Agustine Nengsih, and Mohd N. Norazmi, "Tualang Honey Promotes Apoptotic Cell Death Induced by Tamoxifen in Breast Cancer Cell Lines," *Evidence-Based Complementary and Alternattive Medicine*, (January 2013): 989841, https://www.hindawi.com/journals/ecam/2013/989841/.
5. Sarfraz Ahmed and Nor H. Othman, "The Anti-Cancer Effects of Tualang Honey in Modulating Breast Carcinogenesis: An Experimental Animal Study," *BMC Complementary and Alternative Medicine* 17, no. 1 (April 2017): 208, https://bmccomplementalternmed.biomedcentral.com/articles/10.1186/s12906-017-1721-4.
6. Maria J. Fernandez-Cabezudo et al., "Intravenous Administration of Manuka Honey Inhibits Tumor Growth and Improves Host Survival When Used in Combination with Chemotherapy in a Melanoma Mouse Model," *Public Library of Science One* 8, no. 2 (February 2013): e55993. http://journals.plos .org/plosone/article?id=10.1371/journal.pone.0055993.
7. Noori S. Al-Waili, "Mixture of Honey, Beeswax and Olive Oil Inhibits Growth of *Staphylococcus Aureus* and *Candida Albicans*," *Archives of Medical Research* 36, no. 1 (January 2005): 10–13.
8. Mohammad J. Ansari et al., "Effect of Jujube Honey on *Candida Albicans* Growth and Biofilm Formation," *Archives of Medical Research* 44, no. 5 (July 2013): 352–60.

9. David W. Johnson et al., "Randomized, Controlled Trial of Topical Exit-Site Application of Honey (Medihoney) versus Mupirocin for the Prevention of Catheter-Associated Infections in Hemodialysis Patients," *Journal of the American Society of Nephrology* 16 (February 2005): 1456–62.

10. Fauzi, "Tualang Honey Induces Apoptosis," 871–78.

11. Aamir Shahzad, and Randall J. Cohrs, "In Vitro Antiviral Activity of Honey Against Varicella Zoster Virus (VZV): A Translational Medicine Study for Potential Remedy for Shingles," *Translational Biomedicine* 3, no. 2 (2012), 1–5.

12. Noori S. Al-Waili, "Topical Honey Application vs. Acyclovir for the Treatment of Recurrent Herpes Simplex Lesions," *Medical Science Monitor* 10, no. 8 (2004): MT94-MT98.

13. Rizwana Afroz et al., "Sundarban Honey Confers Protection Against Isoproterenol-Induced Myocardial Infarction in Wistar Rats," *Biomed Research International* 2016: 6437641, https://www.hindawi.com/journals/bmri/2016/6437641/.

14. M. I. Khalil and S. A. Sulaiman, "The Potential Role of Honey and Its Polyphenols in Preventing Heart Diseases: A Review," *African Journal of Traditional, Complementary and Alternative Medicine* 7, no. 4 (2010): 315–21.

15. Ibid.

16. M. E. Octoratou et al, "A Prospective Study of Pre-Illness Diet in Newly Diagnosed Patients with Crohn's Disease." *Revista Medico-Chirurgicala a Societatii De Medici Si Naturalisti Din Iasi* 116, no. 1 (2012): 40–49.

17. Mamdouh Abdulrhman et al., "Metabolic Effects of Honey in Type 1 Diabetes Mellitus: A Randomized Crossover Pilot Study," *Journal of Medicinal Food* 16, no. 1 (January 2013): 66–72.

18. Noori S. Al-Waili, "Intrapulmonary Administration of Natural Honey Solution, Hyperosmolar Dextrose or Hypoosmolar Distill Water to Normal Individuals and to Patients with Type-2 Diabetes Mellitus or Hypertension: Their Effects on Blood Glucose Level, Plasma Insulin and C-Peptide, Blood Pressure and Peaked Expiratory Flow Rate," *European Journal of Medical Research* 8, no. 7 (2003): 295–303.

19. A. Shukrimi, A. R. Sulaiman, A. Y. Halim, and A. Azril, "A Comparative Study Between Honey and Povidone Iodine as Dressing Solution for Wagner Type II Diabetic Foot Ulcers," *Medical Journal of Malaysia* 63, no. 1 (March 2008): 44–46.

20. A. V. Kamaratos et al., "Manuka Honey–Impregnated Dressings in the Treatment of Neuropathic Diabetic Foot Ulcers," *International Wound Journal* 11, no. 3 (June 2014): 259–63.

21. Jennifer J. Eddy, and Mark D. Gideonsen, "Topical Honey for Diabetic Foot Ulcers," *Journal of Family Practice* 54, no. 6 (June 2005): 533–35.

22. Jin-Hyung Lee et al., "Low Concentrations of Honey Reduce Biofilm Formation, Quorum Sensing, and Virulence in *Escherichia Coli* O157:H7," *Biofouling* 27, no. 10 (November 2011): 1095–1104.

23. Adel Alnaqdy et al., "Inhibition Effect of Honey on the Adherence of *Salmonella* to Intestinal Epithelial Cells In Vitro," *International Journal of Food Microbiology* 103, no. 3 (September 2005): 347–51.

24. Berhanu Andualem, "Combined Antibacterial Activity of Stingless Bee (*Apis Mellipodae*) Honey and Garlic (*Allium Sativum*) Extracts against Standard and Clinical Pathogenic Bacteria," *Asian Pacific Journal of Tropical Biomedicine* 3, no. 9 (September 2013): 725–31.

25. Maryam Ekhtelat, Karim Ravaji, and Masood Parvari, "Effect of Iranian Ziziphus Honey on Growth of Some Foodborne Pathogens." *Journal of Natural Science, Biology and Medicine* 7, no. 1 (January 2016): 54–57.

26. Orla Sherlock et al., "Comparison of the Antimicrobial Activity of Ulmo Honey from Chile and Manuka Honey against Methicillin-Resistant *Staphylococcus Aureus, Escherichia Coli* and *Pseudomonas Aeruginosa*," *BMC Complementary and Alternative Medicine* 10 (September 2010): 47, https://bmccomplemental ternmed.biomedcentral.com/articles/10.1186/1472-6882-10-47.

27. Lutfi Tahmaz et al., "Fournier's Gangrene: Report of Thirty-Three Cases and a Review of the Literature," *International Journal Urology* 13, no. 7 (July 2006): 960–67.

28. Fataneh Hashem-Dabaghian, S. Agah, M. Taghavi-Shirazi, and A. Ghobadi, "Combination of *Nigella Sativa* and Honey in Eradication of Gastric *Helicobacter Pylori* Infection," *Iran Red Crescent Medical Journal* 18, no. 11 (November 2016): e23771.

29. Saad B. Almasaudi et al., "Manuka Honey Exerts Antioxidant and Anti-Inflammatory Activities That Promote Healing of Acetic Acid–Induced Gastric Ulcer in Rats," *Evidence-Based Complementary and Alternative Medicine* (January 2017): 5413917, https://www.hindawi.com/journals/ecam /2017/5413917/.

30. Al-Waili, "Topical Honey Application," MT94–MT98.

31. Helen K. P. English, Angela R. C. Pack, and Peter C. Molan, "The Effects of Manuka Honey on Plaque and Gingivitis: A Pilot Study," *Journal of the International Academy of Periodontology* 6, no. 2 (April 2004): 63–67.

32. Al-Dany Atwa, Ramadan Y. AbuShahba, Marwa Mostafa, and Mohamed I. Hashem, "Effect of Honey in Preventing Gingivitis and Dental Caries in Patients Undergoing Orthodontic Treatment," *Saudi Dental Journal* 26, no. 3 (July 2014): 108–14.

33. Ping Zou, "Traditional Chinese Medicine, Food Therapy, and Hypertension Control: A Narrative Review of Chinese Literature," *American Journal of Chinese Medicine* 44, no. 8 (January 2016): 1579–94.

34. Omotayo Erejuwa et al., "Honey Supplementation in Spontaneously Hypertensive Rats Elicits Antihypertensive Effect via Amelioration of Renal Oxidative Stress." *Oxidative Medicine and Cellular Longevity* (2012): 374037, https://www.hindawi.com/journals/omcl/2012/374037/.

35. Mohsen Bahrami et al., "Effects of Natural Honey Consumption in Diabetic Patients: An 8-Week Randomized Clinical Trial," *International Journal of Food Sciences and Nutrition* 60, no. 7 (October 2009): 618–26.

36. Abdulrhman et al., "Metabolic Effects of Honey," 66–72.

37. Noori S. Al-Waili, "An Alternative Treatment for Pityriasis Versicolor, Tinea Cruris, Tinea Corporis and Tinea Faciei with Topical Application of Honey, Olive Oil and Beeswax Mixture: An Open Pilot Study." *Complementary Therapies in Medicine* 12, no. 1 (March 2004): 45–47.

38. Zeina Bassam, Ben I. Zohra, and Al-assad Saada, "The Effects of Honey on *Leishmania* Parasites: An In Vitro Study," *Tropical Doctor* 27, no. 1 (January 1997): 36–38.

39. Fernandez-Cabezudo, "Intravenous Administration of Manuka Honey," e55993.

40. Elena Pichichero et al., "Acacia Honey and Chrysin Reduce Proliferation of Melanoma Cells through Alterations in Cell Cycle Progression," *International Journal of Oncology* 37, no. 4 (October 2010): 973–81.

41. Chunyan Xue et al., "Chrysin Induces Cell Apoptosis in Human Uveal Melanoma Cells via Intrinsic Apoptosis," *Oncology Letters* 12, no. 6 (October 2016): 4813–20.

42. Pradip K. Maiti et al., "The Effect of Honey on Mucositis Induced by Chemoradiation in Head and Neck Cancer," *Journal of the Indian Medical Association* 110, no. 7 (2012): 453–56.

43. Mamdouh Abdulrhman, Nancy S. Elbarbary, Dina Ahmed Amin, and Rania Saeid Ebrahim. 2012. "Honey and a Mixture of Honey, Beeswax, and Olive Oil–Propolis Extract in Treatment of Chemotherapy-Induced Oral Mucositis: A Randomized Controlled Pilot Study," *Pediatric Hematology and Oncology* 29, no. 3 (April 2012): 285–92.

44. B. Khanal, M. Baliga, and N. Uppal, "Effect of Topical Honey on Limitation of Radiation-Induced Oral Mucositis: An Intervention Study," *International Journal of Oral & Maxillofacial Surgery* 39, no. 12 (December 2010): 1181–85.

45. Mohammad A. Raeessi et al., "'Coffee Plus Honey' versus 'Topical Steroid' in the Treatment of Chemotherapy-Induced Oral Mucositis: A Randomised

Controlled Trial," *BMC Complementary and Alternative Medicine* 14 (August 2014): 293, https://bmccomplementalternmed.biomedcentral.com/articles/10.1186/1472-6882-14-293.

46. Darius Henatsch et al., "Treatment of Recurrent Eczematous External Otitis with Honey Eardrops: A Proof-of-Concept Study," *Otolaryngology—Head and Neck Surgery* 157, no. 4 (July 2017): 696–99.

47. Emi Maruhashi et al., "Efficacy of Medical Grade Honey in the Management of Canine Otitis Externa—A Pilot Study," *Veterinary Dermatology* 27, no. 2 (March 2016): 93–e27.

48. Saeed Samarghandian, Jalil T. Afshari, and Saeideh Davoodi, "Chrysin Reduces Proliferation and Induces Apoptosis in the Human Prostate Cancer Cell Line PC-3," *Clinics* (Sao Paulo) 66, no. 6 (2011): 1073–79.

49. R. Cooper, L. Jenkins, and S. Hooper, "Inhibition of Biofilms of *Pseudomonas Aeruginosa* by Medihoney In Vitro." *Journal of Wound Care* 23, no. 3 (March 2014): 93–96, 98–100, 102.

50. R. A. Cooper, E. Halas, and P. C. Molan. 2002. "The Efficacy of Honey in Inhibiting Strains of *Pseudomonas Aeruginosa* from Infected Burns," *Journal of Burn Care & Rehabilitation* 23, no. 6 (November–December 2002): 366–70.

51. Aled E. L. Roberts, Sarah E. Maddocks, and Rose A. Cooper, "Manuka Honey Reduces the Motility of *Pseudomonas Aeruginosa* by Suppression of Flagella-Associated Genes," *Journal of Antimicrobial Chemotherapy* 70, no. 3 (March 2015): 716–25.

52. J. M. Kronda, Rose A. Cooper, and Sarah E. Maddocks, "Manuka Honey Inhibits Siderophore Production in *Pseudomonas Aeruginosa*" *Journal of Applied Microbiology* 115, no. 1 (April 2013): 86–90.

53. Saeed Samarghandian, Jalil T. Afshari, and Saiedeh Davoodi, "Honey Induces Apoptosis in Renal Cell Carcinoma," *Pharmacognosy Magazine* 7, no. 25 (2011): 46–52.

54. Rajendran Mythilypriya, Palanivelu Shanthi, and Panchanadam Sachdanandam, "Synergistic Effect of Kalpaamruthaa on Antiarthritic and Antiinflammatory Properties—Its Mechanism of Action," *Inflammation* 31, no. 6 (December 2008): 391–98.

55. Al-Waili, "An Alternative Treatment," 45–47.

56. Aditya Gupta, Karyn Nicol, and Roma Batra, "Role of Antifungal Agents in the Treatment of Seborrheic Dermatitis," *American Journal of Clinical Dermatology* 5, no. 6 (December 2004): 417–22.

57. Noori S. Al-Waili, "Therapeutic and Prophylactic Effects of Crude Honey on Chronic Seborrheic Dermatitis and Dandruff," *European Journal of Medical Research* 6, no. 7 (August 2001): 306–08.

58. Georgina Gethin and Seamus Cowman, "Bacteriological Changes in Sloughy Venous Leg Ulcers Treated with Manuka Honey or Hydrogel: An RCT," *Journal of Wound Care* 17, no. 6 (June 2008): 241–44, 246–47.

59. Orla Sherlock et al., "Comparison of the Antimicrobial Activity," 47.

60. Talal Alandejani et al., "Effectiveness of Honey on *Staphylococcus Aureus* and *Pseudomonas Aeruginosa* Biofilms," *Otolaryngology—Head and Neck Surgery* 141, no. 1 (July 2009): 114–18.

61. Al-Waili, "An Alternative Treatment," 45–47.

62. Gupta, "Role of Antifungal Agents," 417–22.

63. Bulent Kilicoglu et al., "The Scolicidal Effects of Honey." *Advances in Therapy* 23, no. 6 (November 2006): 1077–83.

64. Yuri V. Efremenko et al., "Clinical Validation of Sublingual Formulations of Immunoxel (Dzherelo) as an Adjuvant Immunotherapy in Treatment of TB Patients," *Immunotherapy* 4, no. 3 (March 2012): 273–82.

65. Ali Akbar Asadi-Pooya, M. R. Pnjehshahin, and S. Beheshti, "The Antimycobacterial Effect of Honey: An In Vitro Study," *Rivista di Biologia* 96, no. 3 (September–December 2003): 491–95.

66. Abdul Hannan, A., Saira Munir, Muhammad U. Arshad, and Nabila Bashir, "In Vitro Antimycobacterial Activity of Pakistani Beri Honey Using BACTEC MGIT 960," *International Scholarly Research Notices*, 2014 (2014): 490589, https://www.hindawi.com/journals/isrn/2014/490589/.

67. Hanaa Z. Nooh and Nermeen M. Nour-Eldien, "The Dual Anti-Inflammatory and Antioxidant Activities of Natural Honey Promote Cell Proliferation and Neural Regeneration in a Rat Model of Colitis," *Acta Histochemica*, 118, no. 6 (July 2016): 588–95.

68. A. Prakash et al., "Effect of Different Doses of Manuka Honey in Experimentally Induced Inflammatory Bowel Disease in Rats," *Phytotherapy Research* 22, no. 11 (August 2008): 1511–19.

69. B. Medhi et al., "Effect of Manuka Honey and Sulfasalazine in Combination to Promote Antioxidant Defense System in Experimentally Induced Ulcerative Colitis Model in Rats." *Indian Journal of Experimental Biology* 46, no. 8 (August 2008): 583–90.

70. Y. Bilsel et al., "Could Honey Have a Place in Colitis Therapy? Effects of Honey, Prednisolone, and Disulfiram on Inflammation, Nitric Oxide, and Free Radical Formation," *Digestive Surgery* 19 (2002): 306–12.

71. Lee et al., "Low Concentrations of Honey Reduce Biofilm Formation," 1095–1104.

72. Somadina Emineke et al., "Diluted Honey Inhibits Biofilm Formation: Potential Application in Urinary Catheter Management?" *Journal of Clinical Pathology* 70, no. 2 (February 2017): 140–44.

73. Nur S. Ahmad, Foong K. Ooi, Mohammed Saat Ismail, and Mahaneem Mohamed, "Effects of Post-Exercise Honey Drink Ingestion on Blood Glucose and Subsequent Running Performance in the Heat." *Asian Journal of Sports Medicine* 6, no. 3 (September 2015): e24044.

74. Peiying Shi et al., "Honey Reduces Blood Alcohol Concentration but Not Affects the Level of Serum MDA and GSH-Px Activity in Intoxicated Male Mice Models," *BMC Complementary and Alternative Medicine* 15 (July 2015): 225, https://bmccomplementalternmed.biomedcentral.com/articles /10.1186/s12906-015-0766-5.

75. Noori S. Al-Waili, Khelod S. Saloom, Thia N. Al-Waili, and Ali N. Al-Waili, "The Safety and Efficacy of a Mixture of Honey, Olive Oil, and Beeswax for the Management of Hemorrhoids and Anal Fissure: A Pilot Study," *Scientific World Journal* 6 (February 2006): 1998–2005.

76. Lynne M. Chepulis, Nicola J. Starkey, Joseph R. Waas, and Peter C. Molan, "The Effects of Long-Term Honey, Sucrose or Sugar-Free Diets on Memory and Anxiety in Rats," *Physiology & Behavior* 97 nos. 3–4 (June 2009): 359–68.

77. Wahab I. Abdulmajeed et al., "Honey Prevents Neurobehavioural Deficit and Oxidative Stress Induced by Lead Acetate Exposure in Male Wistar Rats— A Preliminary Study," *Metabolic Brain Disease* 31, no. 1 (February 2016): 37–44.

78. Badriya Al-Rahbi et al., "Protective Effects of Tualang Honey against Oxidative Stress and Anxiety-Like Behaviour in Stressed Ovariectomized Rats," *International Scholarly Research Notices* 2014 (September 2014): 521065, https://www.hindawi.com/journals/isrn/2014/521065/.

79. Kamran I. Malik, M. A. Malik, and Azhar Aslam, "Honey Compared with Silver Sulphadiazine in the Treatment of Superficial Partial-Thickness Burns," *International Wound Journal* 7, no. 5 (October 2010): 413–17.

80. M. Subrahmanyam, "A Prospective Randomized, Clinical and Histological Study of Superficial Burn Wound Healing with Honey and Silver Sulfadiazine," *Burns* 24, no. 2 (March 1998): 157–61.

81. M. Subrahmanyam, "Topical Application of Honey in Treatment of Burns," *British Journal of Surgery* 78 (1991): 497–98.

82. S. A. El-Haddad, F. Y. Asiri, H. H. Al-Qahtani, and A. S. Al-Ghmlas, "Efficacy of Honey in Comparison to Topical Corticosteroid for Treatment of Recurrent Minor Aphthous Ulceration: A Randomized, Blind, Controlled, Parallel, Double-Center Clinical Trial," *Quintessence International* 45, no. 8 (September 2014): 691–701.

83. Teppei Shibata et al., "Propolis, a Constituent of Honey, Inhibits the Development of Sugar Cataracts and High-Glucose-Induced Reactive

Oxygen Species in Rat Lenses," *Journal of Ophthalmology* 2016 (April 2016): 1917093, https://www.hindawi.com/journals/joph/2016/1917093/.

84. Martin Cernak, Nora Majtanova, Andrej Cernak, and Juraj Majtan, "Honey Prophylaxis Reduces the Risk of Endophthalmitis during Perioperative Period of Eye Surgery," *Phytotherapy Research* 26, no. 4 (October 2011): 613–16.

85. Khairunnuur F. Azman et al., "Tualang Honey Improves Memory Performance and Decreases Depressive-Like Behavior in Rats Exposed to Loud Noise Stress," *Noise Health* 17, no. 75 (March–April 2015): 83–89.

86. Julie M. Albietz and Lee M. Lenton, "Standardised Antibacterial Manuka Honey in the Management of Persistent Post-Operative Corneal Oedema: A Case Series," *Clinical and Experimental Optometry* 98, no. 5 (September 2015): 464–72.

87. Herman A. Cohen et al., "Effect of Honey on Nocturnal Cough and Sleep Quality: A Double-Blind, Randomized, Placebo-Controlled Study," *Pediatrics* 130, no. 3 (September 2012): 465–71.

88. Ian M. Paul et al., "Effect of Honey, Dextromethorphan, and No Treatment on Nocturnal Cough and Sleep Quality for Coughing Children and Their Parents," *Archives of Pediatrics and Adolescent Medicine* 161, no. 12 (2007): 1140–46.

89. Mahmood N. Shadkam, Hassan Mozaffari-Khosravi, and Mohammad R. Mozayan, "A Comparison of the Effect of Honey, Dextromethorphan, and Diphenhydramine on Nightly Cough and Sleep Quality in Children and Their Parents," *Journal of Alternative and Complementary Medicine* 16, no. 7 (July 2010): 787–93.

90. Mohammad A. Raeessi et al., "Honey Plus Coffee versus Systemic Steroid in the Treatment of Persistent Post-Infectious Cough: A Randomised Controlled Trial," *Primary Care Respiratory Journal* 22, no. 3 (August 2013): 325–30.

91. Azman, "Tualang Honey Improves Memory," 83–89.

92. Carlos B. Filho et al., "Chrysin Promotes Attenuation of Depressive-Like Behavior and Hippocampal Dysfunction Resulting from Olfactory Bulbectomy in Mice," *Chemico-Biological Interactions* 260 (December 2016): 154–62.

93. Noori S. Al-Waili, "Clinical and Mycological Benefits of Topical Application of Honey, Olive Oil and Beeswax in Diaper Dermatitis," *Clinical Microbiology and Infection* 11, no. 2 (February 2005): 160–63.

94. Mamdouh A. Abdulrhman, Mohamed A. Mekawy, Maha M. Awadalla, and Ashraf H. Mohamed, "Bee Honey Added to the Oral Rehydration Solution in

Treatment of Gastroenteritis in Infants and Children," *Journal of Medicinal Food* 13, no. 3 (June 2010): 605–09.

95. Daniel Wong et al., "Treatment of Contact Lens Related Dry Eye with Antibacterial Honey," *Contact Lens & Anterior Eye* 40, no. 6 (December 2017): 389–93.

96. Julie M. Albietz and Lee M. Lenton, "Effect of Antibacterial Honey on the Ocular Flora in Tear Deficiency and Meibomian Gland Disease." *Cornea* 25, no. 9 (October 2006): 1012–19.

97. Noori S. Al-Waili, "Topical Application of Natural Honey, Beeswax and Olive Oil Mixture for Atopic Dermatitis or Psoriasis: Partially Controlled, Single-Blinded Study," *Complementary Therapies in Medicine* 11, no. 4 (December 2003): 226–34.

98. Noori Al-Waili et al.,."Synergistic Effects of Honey and Propolis Toward Drug Multi-Resistant *Staphylococcus Aureus, Escherichia Coli* and *Candida Albicans* Isolates in Single and Polymicrobial Cultures," *International Journal of Medical Sciences* 9, no. 9 (2012): 793–800.

99. Alandejani et al., "Effectiveness of Honey," 114–18.

100. Mahmoud Ebrahimi et al., "Effects of Dietary Honey and Ardeh Combination on Chemotherapy-Induced Gastrointestinal and Infectious Complications in Patients with Acute Myeloid Leukemia: A Double-Blind Randomized Clinical Trial," *Iranian Journal of Pharmaceutical Research* 15, no. 2 (Spring 2016): 661–68.

101. Ken Watanabe et al., "Anti-Influenza Viral Effects of Honey In Vitro: Potent High Activity of Manuka Honey," *Archives of Medical Research* 45, no. 5 (July 2014): 359–65.

102. Ibid.

103. Al-Waili et al., "The Safety and Efficacy of a Mixture," 1998–2005.

104. Ahmed Abdelhafiz and Jehan A. Muhamad, "Midcycle Pericoital Intravaginal Bee Honey and Royal Jelly for Male Factor Infertility," *International Journal of Gynecology & Obstetrics* 101, no. 2 (January 2008): 146–49.

105. Saba Z. Hussein, Kamaruddin Mohd Yusoff, Suzana Makpol, and Yasmin A. Mohd Yusof, "Gelam Honey Inhibits the Production of Proinflammatory, Mediators NO, PGE(2), TNF-α, and IL-6 in Carrageenan-Induced Acute Paw Edema in Rats," *Evidence-Based Complementary and Alternative Medicine* 2012 (2012): 109636, https://www.hindawi.com/journals/ecam/2012/109636/.

106. W. A. Nijhuis, R. H. Houwing, W. C. Van der Zwet, and F. G. Jansman, "A Randomised Trial of Honey Barrier Cream versus Zinc Oxide Ointment," *British Journal of Nursing* 21, no. sup20 (2012): S10-S13.

107. Abdulmajeed et al., "Honey Prevents Neurobehavioural Deficit and Oxidative Stress," 37–44.

108. Erejuwa, "Honey Supplementation in Spontaneously Hypertensive Rats," 374037.

109. Karsten Münstedt et al., "Bee Pollen and Honey for the Alleviation of Hot Flushes and Other Menopausal Symptoms in Breast Cancer Patients," *Molecular and Clinical Oncology* 3, no. 4 (July 2015): 869–74.

110. Zahiruddin Othman et al., "Improvement in Immediate Memory after 16 Weeks of Tualang Honey (Agro Mas) Supplement in Healthy Postmenopausal Women," *Menopause* 18, no. 11 (November 2011): 1219–24.

111. Siti S. M. Zaid, Siti A. Sulaiman, Kuttulebbai N. M. Sirajudeen, and Nor H. Othman, "The Effects of Tualang Honey on Female Reproductive Organs, Tibia Bone and Hormonal Profile in Ovariectomised Rats—Animal Model for Menopause," *BMC Complementary and Alternative Medicine* 10 (December 2010): 82, https://bmccomplementalternmed.biomedcentral.com /articles/10.1186/1472-6882-10-82.

112. Noori S. Al-Waili, "Investigating the Antimicrobial Activity of Natural Honey and Its Effects on the Pathogenic Bacterial Infections of Surgical Wounds and Conjunctiva," *Journal of Medicinal Food* 7, no. 2 (2004): 210–22.

113. Alex A. Ilechie et al., "The Efficacy of Stingless Bee Honey for the Treatment of Bacteria-Induced Conjunctivitis in Guinea Pigs," *Journal of Experimental Pharmacology* 4 (2012): 63–68.

114. Al-Waili, "Topical Application of Natural Honey," 226–34.

115. Abdulrhman et al., "Bee Honey Added to the Oral Rehydration Solution," 605–09.

116. Ahmad et al., "Effects of Post-Exercise Honey Drink," e24044.

117. Irene Braithwaite et al., "Randomised Controlled Trial of Topical Kanuka Honey for the Treatment of Rosacea." *BMJ Open* 5, no. 6 (June 2015): e007651, http://bmjopen.bmj.com/content/5/6/e007651.

118. K. Saarinen, J. Jantunen, and T. Haahtela, "Birch Pollen Honey for Birch Pollen Allergy—A Randomized Controlled Pilot Study," *International Archives of Allergy and Immunology* 155, no. 2 (May 2011): 160–66.

119. Zamzil A, Asha'ari et al., "Ingestion of Honey Improves the Symptoms of Allergic Rhinitis: Evidence from a Randomized Placebo-Controlled Trial in the East Coast of Peninsular Malaysia," *Annals of Saudi Medicine* 33, no. 5 (2013): 469–75.

120. Alandejani, T., "Effectiveness of Honey," 114–18.

121. F. Hashemian et al., "The Effect of Thyme Honey Nasal Spray on Chronic Rhinosinusitis: A Double-Blind Randomized Controlled Clinical Trial." *European Archives of Oto-Rhino-Laryngology* 272, no. 6 (June 2015): 1429–35.

122. Sanna Huttunen, Kaisu Riihinen, Jussi Kauhanen, and Carina Tikkanen-Kaukanen, "Antimicrobial Activity of Different Finnish Monofloral Honeys against Human Pathogenic Bacteria," *APMIS* 121, no. 9 (September 2013): 827–34.

123. Sarah E. Maddocks et al., "Manuka Honey Inhibits Adhesion and Invasion of Medically Important Wound Bacteria In Vitro." *Future Microbiology* 8, no. 12 (December 2013): 1523–36.

124. Samet Ozlugedik et al.,"Can Postoperative Pains Following Tonsillectomy Be Relieved by Honey? A Prospective, Randomized, Placebo Controlled Preliminary Study," *International Journal of Pediatric Otorhinolaryngology* 70, no. 11 (November 2006): 1929–34.

125. Norhafiza Mat Lazim, Baharudin Abdullah, and Rosdan Salim, "The Effect of Tualang Honey in Enhancing Post Tonsillectomy Healing Process. An Open Labelled Prospective Clinical Trial." *International Journal of Pediatric Otorhinolaryngology* 77, no. 4 (April 2013): 457–61.

126. Baharudin Abdullah, Norhafiza M. Lazim, and Rosdan Salim, "The Effectiveness of Tualang Honey in Reducing Post-tonsillectomy Pain," *The Turkish Journal of Ear Nose and Throat* 25, no. 3 (2015): 137–43.

127. Atwa et al., "Effect of Honey in Preventing Gingivitis and Dental Caries," 108–14.

128. S. Rupesh et al., "Evaluation of the Effects of Manuka Honey on Salivary Levels of *Mutans Streptococci* in Children: A Pilot Study," *Journal of Indian Society Pedodontics and Preventive Dentistry* 32, no. 3 (July–September 2014): 212–19.

129. Abdulrhman et al., "Bee Honey Added to the Oral Rehydration Solution," 605–09.

130. D. E. Larson-Meyer et al., "Effect of Honey versus Sucrose on Appetite, Appetite-Regulating Hormones, and Postmeal Thermogenesis," *Journal of the American College of Nutrition* 29, no. 5 (2010): 482–93.

131. Tricia M. Nemoseck et al., "Honey Promotes Lower Weight Gain, Adiposity, and Triglycerides than Sucrose in Rats." *Nutrition Research* 31, no. 1 (January 2011): 55–60.

132. R. F. Ingle, R., J. B. Levin, and K. Polinder, "Wound Healing with Honey—A Randomised Controlled Trial," *South African Medical Journal* 96, no. 9 (2006): 831–85.

133. Ülkü Yapucu Günes and Ismet Eser, "Effectiveness of a Honey Dressing for Healing Pressure Ulcers," *Journal of Wound, Ostomy and Continence Nursing* 34, no. 2 (March–April 2007): 184–90.

134. Aykut Misirlioglu et al., "Use of Honey as an Adjunct in the Healing of Split-Thickness Skin Graft Donor Site," *Dermatologic Surgery* 29, no. 2 (February 2003): 168–72.

135. Betina Lund-Nielsen et al., "The Effect of Honey-Coated Bandages Compared with Silver-Coated Bandages on Treatment of Malignant Wounds—A Randomized Study," *Wound Repair and Regeneration* 19, no. 6 (November 2011): 664–70.

136. Georgina Gethin and Seamus Cowman, "Case Series of Use of Manuka Honey in Leg Ulceration," *International Wound Journal* 2, no. 1 (March 2005): 10–15.

137. Elin Julianti, Kasturi Rajah, and Irda Fidrianny, "Antibacterial Activity of Ethanolic Extract of Cinnamon Bark, Honey, and Their Combination Effects against Acne-Causing Bacteria," *Scientia Pharmaceutica* 85, no. 2 (2017), pii-e19.

138. Nan-Lin Wu et al., "Chrysin Protects Epidermal Keratinocytes from UVA- and UVB-Induced Damage," *Journal of Agricultural and Food Chemistry* 59, no. 15 (2011): 8391–8400.

139. Israr Ahmad, Hugo Jimenez, Nik S. Yaacob, and Nabiha Yusuf, "Tualang Honey Protects Keratinocytes from Ultraviolet Radiation–Induced Inflammation and DNA Damage," *Photochemistry and Photobiology* 88, no. 5 (September–October 2012): 1198–1204.

140. Al-Waili, "Therapeutic and Prophylactic Effects of Crude Honey," 306–308.

141. Julianti et al., "Antibacterial Activity," p11–e19.

142. Braithwaite, "Randomised Controlled Trial of Topical Kanuka Honey," e007651.

143. Ahmad, "Tualang Honey Protects Keratinocytes," 1198–1204.

ABOUT THE AUTHOR

SUSAN BRANSON earned an undergraduate degree in biology from St. Francis Xavier University and then an MS in toxicology from the University of Ottawa. From there, she worked in research: in the field, in the lab, as a writer, and as an administrator. She took time off to stay at home after her second child was born. In addition to being a stay-at-home mom, she also took violin lessons, took photography courses, earned a diploma in writing, and ultimately became a holistic nutritional consultant. Susan is a member of the alumni association of the Canadian School of Natural Nutrition (CSNN), Canada's leading holistic nutrition school.

AB0UT FAMILIUS

VISIT 0UR WEBSITE: WWW.FAMILIUS.COM

JOIN 0UR FAMILY

There are lots of ways to connect with us! Subscribe to our newsletters at www.familius.com to receive uplifting daily inspiration, essays from our Pater Familius, a free ebook every month, and the first word on special discounts and Familius news.

GET BULK DISCOUNTS

If you feel a few friends and family might benefit from what you've read, let us know and we'll be happy to provide you with quantity discounts. Simply email us at orders@familius.com.

CONNECT

Facebook: www.facebook.com/paterfamilius
Twitter: @familiustalk, @paterfamilius1
Pinterest: www.pinterest.com/familius
Instagram: @familiustalk

THE M0ST IMPORTANT W0RK Y0U EVER D0 WILL BE WITHIN THE WALLS OF Y0UR 0WN HOME.

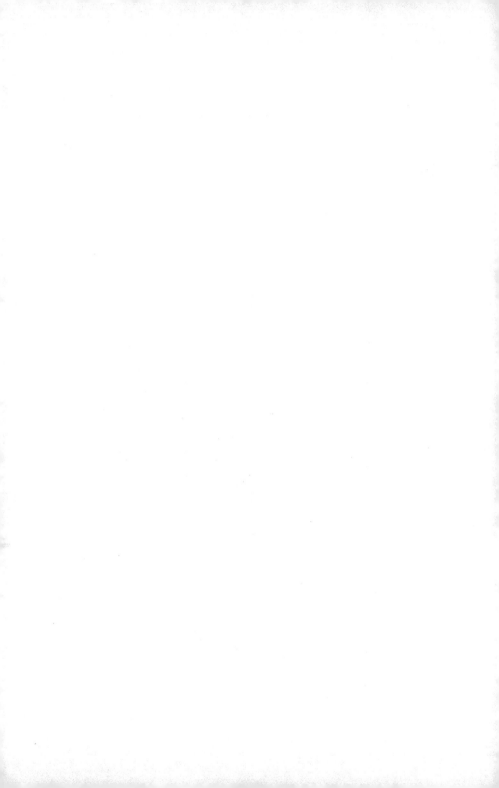

CPSIA information can be obtained
at www.ICGtesting.com
Printed in the USA
FSHW022307281218

9 781641 700443